"The complex universe of human hormones comes to life in this book. Dr. Kryger presents a rational and comprehensive overview of the male hormones."

—André Guay, endocrinologist
Lahey Clinic, Harvard University

"Dr. Kryger's book is exactly what people need to read. I especially like the patient examples, which add life and 'a face' to this disorder from which they suffer alone in silence. This is a hormone guidebook for everyone. Very clear and concise explanation of the action of hormones on the brain."

—Leslie Lunt, MD, psychiatrist
author of Think Like a Psychiatrist

"Easy to understand, up-to-date, well researched approach to a difficult subject."

—Howard Wynne, MD
clinical professor, UCLA School of Medicine

"This is a must-have reference for every man who wants to be happier and healthier. Using the latest medical evidence as its inspiration, the book cuts through the hype and confusion about one of the most misunderstood aspects of men's health, the vital role of testosterone and other hormones. I recommend this fascinating book to all my clients with sexual dysfunction."

—Evelyn Waterman, PhD, psychotherapist
Santa Monica, California

"This book contains a wealth of information and provides practical ways that men can begin to rebalance their hormones and rebuild their health. Recent research is making it increasingly clear that many middle-aged and older men could benefit from supplemental bio-identical testosterone."

—John Robbins
'hor of Diet for a New America

A WOMAN'S GUIDE TO MEN'S HEALTH

ABRAHAM HARVEY KRYGER, MD, DMD

RDR Books
Berkeley • Muskegon

A Woman's Guide to Men's Health

RDR Books
1487 Glen Ave.
Muskegon, MI 49441
Phone: (510) 595-0595
Fax: (510) 228-0300
E-mail: read@rdrbooks.com
www.rdrbooks.com

ISBN: 1-57143-156-X
After Jan. 1, 2007: 978-1-57143-156-1

Library of Congress Control Number: 2006921008

Design and Production: Richard Harris

Distributed in the United Kingdom and Europe by
Roundhouse Publishing Ltd., Millstone, Limers Lane,
Northam, North Devon EX39 2RG, United Kingdom

Printed in Canada

CONTENTS

INTRODUCTION

Recently I published a book titled *Listen To Your Hormones (especially for men)*. I was astonished and delighted by the response from all over the world. Many who wrote to thank me for explaining, for the first time, the vital role the endocrine system plays in their health. The number of women who felt the same way also surprised me.

"Thank you Doctor, this is the book I have been looking for and I am giving it to my husband tonight," wrote one. Another responded by arriving at my office with her husband in tow. I began receiving calls from men who had been referred by women who had just finished my book. Some told me they didn't think they needed help and then went on to confide that their partner had insisted they make an appointment.

After finishing *Listen To Your Hormones*, many women wrote and phoned me with specific questions. Many of them wanted to know how they could educate their husbands on a proven and painless way to restore their health. This book, *A Woman's Guide to Men's Health*, answers those important questions and provides a simple course of action that can show women how to effectively care for their partner's health and avoid chronic illness.

Men have put themselves in jeopardy by ignoring their health, smoking too much and eating a punishing diet while drinking to excess, failing to exercise and not protecting themselves against environmental toxins. Compounding the problem is the fact that men tend to ignore valuable sources of information and are reluctant to visit a doctor to head off serious medical problems.

Men feel emotion as much as women but do not deal with it openly. Men need to be educated that feeling emotion is healthy and not a sign of weakness. That's why I wrote this book. To help men understand their bodies.

Based on thirty years of research and clinical practice, I have tried to provide some answers and strategies for dealing with these issues. Before we go any further, I want you to understand that books are not a substitute for visiting your personal physician.

Even though sexuality is extremely important to their patients, physicians often do not introduce the subject during visits nor do they address sexual concerns with patients. This is because professional training in sexual health is limited. Without some physician prompting, patients are reluctant to bring up sexual concerns. This is a significant problem for our patients. Sexual dysfunction affects over 40 million women and 30 million men; about one quarter of our population and it often goes untreated.

Indeed the first step in improving your health or that of your husband or partner is finding an open-minded doctor. If you don't have a physician experienced in hormone prescribing, you can call or email me for suggestions on how to find a good doctor in your area.

With this book in hand, your spouse can work closely with his doctor to come up with a sensible plan based on the latest medical research. The first step is to make that appointment and get tested for hormonal imbalances. No, this is not about popping Viagra or some other self-styled "miracle drug" that merely provides symptomatic relief. Rather it's about coming up with a comprehensive plan that includes the appropriate medication, a healthier diet plan, exercise plus the elimination of toxic substances like fast foods, alcohol and cigarettes.

Once the man in your life has begun the process essential to restoring his well being, he is well on his way to improved health. If he is reluctant to make that appointment, simply tell him what you are learning from reading this book. When you find a case study about a patient with a similar problem, he will probably grab it out of your hands. As this is a book about wellness, you will appreciate the fact that my focus is both on disease prevention and treatment with bioidentical hormones.

Hormones play a major role in sexual difficulties. All too often, the problem is a malfunction of the endocrine system. For example, the section on anabolic steroids is critical reading for your sons and daughters, especially if they are active in sports.

One of the questions men often ask me is "why is my wife constantly bugging me to see you or my doctor?" Typically, a first-time patient said, "I didn't even want to come here but my wife thinks I need to see you. What's this all about?" The primary obstacle is patient inaction, unwillingness for men to admit that anything is wrong or that they need help. This attitude has been programmed into their psyche as they grow up.

When a new patient telephoned after reading my book and said, "My wife and I read your book over the weekend and realized that we both need to come to see you," I felt as if I had done my job. He went on to clarify, "So many of the patients you describe mirror our problems. We're so excited to know that there's help and that there are other patients like us. Now we don't have to wait any longer to find an answer."

It's common knowledge that women pay much closer attention to hormonal imbalances than men. Everybody knows that women outlive men, but did you know why? Bookstores are filled with numerous titles about women's hormones. Women spend billions on prescriptions for products like Premarin®, Climara® or Provera® to treat hormonal imbalances. Try and find comparable books for men and you won't find them. It's also true that when men do go to the doctor they are quicker to focus on a symptom like pain than they are on their overall health.

Women know all about the consequences of hormone use in their own lives because they read books about it, visit their doctors, take hormone replacement therapies and follow up with their doctors. Unfortunately, men do not, nor do they take advantage of the advances concerning them in the field of endocrinology.

A woman's concern for her man is based on the fact that she already knows more about hormones than he does. Most men think that male hormones are associated with sexuality, aggression, moodiness and violent behavior, but what they don't know is that ignorance about their hormones, chiefly testosterone, creates more damage to their health. This book can act as a guide to help women ask the important questions that will convince their partners to visit a doctor. The doctor will then help you determine if the answers involve hormonal deficiencies.

Unfortunately, low testosterone is only one of many undiagnosed crises that both men and women face. Men have problems with obesity more often than women, who have depression more often than testosterone deficiency. But that doesn't make any one of these health risks less important. These are a few of the numerous problems caused by a malfunctioning hormone system: memory loss, decreased libido and increased weight, along with depression and laziness or inability to help around the house. Moreover your husband may also experience: sleep problems, increased appetite, snoring and a diminished sexual arousal. In addition, your spouse may lose his morning erections; notice a lack of interest in any contact—including cuddling and kissing.

In this book you will learn why your husband is tired all the time.

Why he comes home, plops down in front of the TV and is too bushed to cut the grass. Why he doesn't seem to have any energy left for you. He just doesn't seem like the guy you married. Perhaps he has even lost interest in sex and is grumpy all the time. You will learn why he doesn't think there is anything wrong. You will learn how smoking, drinking, environmental pollution and a bad diet can cause hormonal imbalances in anyone. Yet it is our lifestyles and the world around us that seem to contribute the most damaging, long-lasting poisons to our bodies.

I will discuss some of these poisons in great detail to help you find solutions to your concerns. My motivation, my passion if you will, is to educate you—men and women, young and old alike—on the need for hormonal balance, in terms of both your sexual health and your health in general.

Although I have been in clinical practice for many years writing for a popular audience is a true labor of love. It is one thing to have a patient come in after months of treatment and report that their medical problem has been explained. It is quite another to have readers from around the world report that they have taken your book to their own doctors, seeking important treatment they have avoided for years.

This book is based on the principle that all of us, doctors, patients and their partners, need to take better care of our hormones because they are vital to our good health. You'll also learn the truth, free of any propaganda from the drug companies, about your hormones and how they regulate your sexual performance. But this book is more than a quick fix. In fact, this book is about a lot more than sex.

While my book is primarily focused on male health problems, it will also present information for women on testosterone, including the new age-specific levels of sex hormones for women. This will enable medical doctors to diagnose and treat female hormone deficiencies more accurately. If you work with your physician, together we can solve this intricate problem.

This book will become a valuable resource that you will refer to again and again. By all means, feel free to share this information with your personal physician. Once again, your doctor is the ideal person to help you or the man in your life to good health. Consult with him or her before embarking on any health plan. They will walk you both through the tests crucial to assessing the health of your hormonal systems and then prescribe a treatment plan that makes sense. I dedicate *A Woman's Guide to Men's Health* to your doctor, those men who are interested in their health and the women who love them.

1

YOUR HORMONES:
THE DRIVING FORCE

Hormones, the Language of the Body

Male or female, nothing in the universe exceeds the power of our hormones. From the instant we were conceived, our hormones have been driving our body and influencing our every thought. Without hormones, life as we know it could not exist. Without hormones, we would never feel a longing for sex or a thousand other desires.

Remember the excitement you felt the first time you sensed that you were in love? You were electrified, stupefied and confused! Your heart beat faster. Perhaps touching the hand of your romantic interest made you feel light-headed and sweaty. You may have found yourself talking endlessly to friends about this incredible person. Maybe you began sending them loving notes. Your parents may have kidded that you were a victim of "raging hormones."

While people joke easily about hormones, my clinical experience suggests that most people don't know much about how hormones influence their daily lives. Hormonal impulses spring forth at childbirth, instantly bonding the mother to her newborn baby. A hormonal burst emerges from the father's brain to create a permanent paternal relationship with the infant. Of course, the same hormones also establish a lifelong link between a mother and her child.

Hormones are biological messengers that speak the language of the human body. Hormones drive us to do things we never imagined possible. A passing glance or a faint scent can arouse our hormones, triggering feelings that lead to a passion for love or sex. They ignore our inhibitions. The sight of your child sliding off the bank into a raging river turns your muscles into steel as adrenaline empowers you to perform superhuman feats. You're drowsy at work because your brain has too much melatonin, a hormone that senses light, or you're up at midnight raiding the refrigerator because you don't have enough of this same hormone. Yes, it's true that hormones control your appetite, your sleep patterns and your sex drive as well as your way of thinking.

What are these mysterious forces that disrupt the calm and logical way we view our world? Do they force us to make bad decisions? Would the quality of our lives improve if our hormones didn't influence us in so many ways? The fact is that we couldn't survive without them. Hormones affect how every cell and system in our body functions. They control our brain's ability to regulate everything we say, think and do. They direct all bodily functions, in addition to our behavior.

Hormones are essential to life and converse with each other and our brains while simultaneously carrying messages throughout our body. These tiny hormone messengers act as the on-off switch for our genes by setting different production levels for the manufacturing of proteins or enzymes. Some hormones are secreted at a steady rate and others in spurts, repeating every few minutes or each 24 hours. As an example, hormones that produce the menstrual cycle rise and fall throughout the month; some hormones may cycle with the seasons and others are only secreted in emergencies.

Our bodies host eight miniature hormone-producing factories or "glands" located in strategic positions: the pituitary and the pineal gland in our brain, the thyroid in our throat, the thymus in the upper chest area, the adrenals and the pancreas near the kidneys. Protected by the pelvic bones, the female ovaries and the male testes produce our sex hormones. Some glands do double duty, for example, the pancreas, known for the insulin hormone, also releases chemicals that help us to digest our food. The adrenal glands generate cortisol and dehydroepiandrosterone or DHEA. Our sex organs produce multiple hormones including testosterone, estrogen and progesterone. Vital organs such as the brain, lungs, heart, kidneys, liver, skin and digestive tract also manufacture hormones, though that is not their primary function. Hormones endow our bodies with an efficient communication system.

In amounts as tiny as a thousandth, a millionth, or a trillionth of a gram, hormones travel at lightning speed in your blood to reach targeted cells. After an immediate match, the hormones direct your body's organs and genes to do their job: inducing an emotion or a behavior and performing an essential life function while releasing more hormones.

Taken together, these hormone-producing organs are known as the endocrine system. Doctors who specialize in hormone function and treat people with hormone problems are called endocrinologists. Endocrinology specialists who focus on male hormones or androgens are termed andrologists. Because there are so many vital hormones, endocrinologists usually focus on one or two hormones, at the most, plus the specific diseases related to those hormones.

Hormones originate from secreting cells in the endocrine glands and enter our bloodstream directly. For example, hormones from the pituitary gland in our brain bind to receptors in our thyroid, triggering the immediate release of thyroid hormones. In tiny amounts hormones traverse our entire body in less than a second. If the pituitary senses that there is already too much thyroid hormone in our system, it cuts back its stimulation in a process known as *negative feedback*. We will call on this concept often in relation to the endocrine system.

Hormones operate an intricate command center more complex than the systems that control robots on Mars. Your hormones turn your genes on and off. They work like a power switch, signaling your genes to start up the processes that make specific proteins in the miniature protein factories or ribosomes, inside your body's cells. Your hormones circulate all over your body, performing a fantastic set of signaling and triggering routines. No computer can operate with the self-regulating and self-repairing efficiency of your endocrine system.

The master control system of the pituitary and pineal gland plus the hypothalamus is called the *neurohypophysis*. These three brain structures govern the formation and release of many nerve hormones. A short list would have to include melatonin, oxytocin, testosterone, estrogen, progesterone and vasopressin. Others in this category activate substances known as hormone releasing factors or *neurohormones*. This interesting class of hormones, created in the brain's control center, serves as transmitting or switching devices.

While most other hormones originate in our endocrine system and circulate to reach target cells, certain hormones like the neurohormones originate from specific brain cells we call *neurons*. They can travel to their destination in our blood, via the fluid of our brain and spinal column, or they can diffuse into the spaces between cells of our nervous system. Some neurohormones travel along nerves directly to the pituitary gland where they are stored and then released. Neurohormones are also referred to as *neurosteroids*.

This brain language control center, the *neurohypophysis* secretes neurosteroids that subsequently affect the endocrine system by triggering a variety of hormone releases. The amazing consequences of these connections are sure to fascinate anyone who wants to know how their brain works. Whether you realize it or not, neurohormones affect the way your mind controls everything in your body, from moment to moment both day and night. Neurohormones are not only responsible for the amazing changes that occur in your body as you grow from child to adult, but they also influence hunger, thirst, sleep and blood pressure as well as perspiration along with thrills and chills.

I know you want to hear about the thrills and chills part, but first we should talk about the basic words of this hormone language. As you read, I will add additional information so that you can begin to appreciate the basics of this complex communication system.

When we first learn to speak, most of us mimic sounds we hear made by those around us. Think of hormones as mimics that can absorb any word or concept immediately and understand it within microseconds. This book will teach you not only how hormones work but also what can disrupt or upset their exquisite balance.

This awareness of the balance of our bodies allows hormones to keep us in tune. Hormones allow us to maintain a sense of well-being, that feeling that everything is fine and good. From day to day hormones determine most of our behavior. All of our hormones must function in perfect harmony in order for us to enjoy good health and normal sexual function, but that delicate balance of neurotransmitters and hormones can become disrupted in a flash. What could disrupt our neurohormones? Read on!

Does Sex Follow a Rhythm or a Whim?

Hormonal rhythms and genetics control our sexual behavior leading to the creation of new life through conception and pregnancy. As we grow into physical maturity, impulses and instincts make us long for an intimate relationship, guiding us on the path to sexual fulfillment. Simply put, we are born, we grow up and have children, hopefully staying in love and feeling contented till we breathe our last breath. This cycle of life is idyllic but it is not always perfect. We do not all necessarily achieve healthy sexual functioning.

Biology and behavior interact with numerous psychosocial factors to permit you to experience healthy sexual functioning. What does that mean? You encompass a complex being dependant on your nervous system, heart and hormonal coordination, which is in turn influenced by your family and religious background, your sexual partner and individual factors such as your self-concept and self-esteem.

A wide variety of natural incentives including self-respect, your body image and your relationship with your sexual partner are essential for a person to initiate or be receptive to sexual activity. For women, touch and loving words together with a stable relationship are of greater import; for men visual stimuli are all that's needed. Are these behaviors inherent or learned?

Nature versus nurture has been a common theme in human research and both factors are crucial. In her book *Sex On The Brain*, Deborah Blum said, "We can choose to override an instinct… Think of biology and behavior as dancers—one leads, the other follows. But which does which and when? They tug at each other and in turn are pulled by the music, the fluid melody of the environment and do we ever know—can we ever know—where we are in the dance?" It seems that nature and nurture interact to form our behaviors.

What drives the behaviors that create these dances, as Blum calls them? It all begins with your genetic code. Every living organism owns a unique set of genes made of DNA, the coded information or blueprint for life. Human chromosomes are coiled units of DNA with 22 identical pairs plus one set of sex chromosomes per person. They are located within the nucleus or center of every cell and determine the formation of each organ, tissue and cell in your body.

Before you were born your body carried one X chromosome from your mother and an additional chromosome that could be either an X or a Y from your father. If the second chromosome happened to be a Y, you would be born as a male. An XX chromosome pair meant you would be a female. Early life forms did not contain any sex chromosomes because these organisms had no need for sexual reproduction. As animals evolved, the two X chromosomes mutated until eventually one of them developed in a way that caused the male and female sexes to emerge.

The Y chromosome therefore was the result of a 300 million-year experiment. Some of the X chromosome's genes were deleted and new functions were added as the Y chromosome became more and more specialized in the evolving mammals. The Y chromosome shrank and added the testes gene to manufacture and store sperm and at that point males were created as different from females.

Yes, it seems that at one point all life forms were female and able to reproduce without the need for sexual differentiation or males. All offspring were identical to the female mother much like *clones*. Once there was a separation of the sexes, evolution created a line of males and females who are quite different from each other and yet belong to the same species. The genetic code is the blueprint that makes you unique and independent.

The X chromosome has about two thousand genes, while the Y chromosome has a few dozen; so much for superiority of the male. Females have redundant genes or spare parts, which may explain why they outlive men. Our sex chromosomes do far more than merely determine whether we will be male or female. The way we look, the color of our eyes and hair and various physical and psychological features of each parent are passed on to us by our chromosomes. The level and functionality of our sex hormones and possibly our sexual preference are all under the domain of these powerful DNA molecules, called *genes*.

In addition to genes, hormones are intimately connected to human development. The circadian rhythms, the name we give to the 24-hour hormonal cycles based on the light-dark sequences, regulate our hormones and are deeply embedded in our brain. Cycles are common in Nature. Winter turns into spring, spring to summer; night becomes day. These changes in nature are known as biocycles and our brains and hormones are set to follow them. This timing of life is present in all animals, insects and plants. Flies also have a sleep-awake cycle, which is why we can sneak up on them while they're sitting on the ceiling or wall. They're sound asleep!

At this point you should realize that cycles and hormones go hand in hand. The endocrine system has evolved over millions of years to allow you to respond to your environment and survive. Yet, this system is exquisitely sensitive to changes in the environment. You don't have to travel into space or descend deep into a mine for something to drastically upset your ingrained cycle of day and night. In any situation where light and darkness do not vary on a predicable 24-hour basis, you can experience a disruption of your inherent sense of your own cycle. In as little as three weeks, this imbalance can become noticeable. Sleeping less than six hours a night can increase your appetite and make you sleepy during the daytime. Sleeping more than nine hours could be a sign of depression.

Some night-shift workers complain of daytime fatigue because they have forced themselves to stay awake at night when their bodies wanted to sleep. Nurses on night shift, firemen, security guards, doctors and police officers often work during the night but they are able to adjust their circadian rhythms according to their schedules. This does take time to adapt. Other people are genuine "night owls" and do not feel alert until midnight because their bodies have modified their biocycles for a reverse dark-light sequence.

If they get a day job, people with this condition drag themselves through the day and lie awake at night. This cycle variation results in too little sleep, which robs them of the energy needed to deal well with the next day's activities and may contribute to hormonal imbalances and increased hunger. A similar effect arises when people with a normal circadian rhythm must stay awake at night. The next day, feeling sluggish but ravenous, they have trouble remembering things and constantly try to fall asleep. This same response occurs in many mammals.

Among all mammals hormonal cycles determine the way seasonal changes trigger mating or territorial aggression. Mating hormones are released at peak intensity, or, as we say, when the animals are "in heat" and ready to mate. Healthy humans, on the other hand, can mate any time they choose, without regard to nature's seasons or the time of day. On some level this might give rise to problems since most people are not sensitive to their hormonal cycles. Sexual difficulties among couples often result from this hormonal insensitivity.

If you lack a full, satisfying sexual relationship, you are not alone. If you add the estimated 30 million men with erectile dysfunction, to the estimated 13 million men with testosterone deficiency and include the 40 million women suffering some degree of sexual dysfunction, we are talking about one third of the American population. In 2003 according to the Massachusetts Male Aging Study, 52 percent of men over the age of 40 had some degree of erectile failure.

Are millions struggling with a sexual disorder while the rest of the country is enjoying good sex? I doubt it; there are varying degrees of satisfaction and compromise when it comes to relationships. Still it is rather disheartening, isn't it? If your husband or lover is not interested in sex and he is irritable much of the time, you are not alone!

What is The Irritable Male Syndrome?

Is it possible that low hormones can affect our moods? Yes, Irritable Male Syndrome (IMS) is a common condition, occurring in men when their hormone levels drop, either because of age or for other reasons. Men may blame their discomfort on retirement or problems at work, but anyone with constant hot flashes would feel depressed. The hormone problems that cause men to feel depressed fade in comparison with what some women endure.

Irritable Male Syndrome is taken from the better-known premenstrual syndrome (PMS) that makes women irritable and bloated. By the way, recent evidence has surfaced from an ongoing Nurse's Health Study that women who had the lowest levels of vitamin D and calcium-rich foods had the highest risk of PMS. The authors concluded that these two food substances were effective treatments for the symptoms of PMS. Those women consuming at least 1200 milligrams of calcium and 400 IU of vitamin D were less likely to experience irritability, fatigue, stomach cramps or mood disorders before their monthly period.

One of my patients, who could not figure out why his wife said, "You act like you have PMS," asked me if men ever get PMS. I thought about this for a while and responded as follows:

Jed Diamond writes extensively of the psychological problems in men as they age in his new book, *The Irritable Male Syndrome*, "Men afflicted with irritable male syndrome become grumpy, depressed and lose self-esteem. Sexual desire declines. Interest in work and career diminishes. Living hardly seems worthwhile." He goes far beyond this quote to offer user-friendly advice for coping. I recommend you read Jed's other books on male menopause as well.

The primary cause of the irritable male syndrome implicates a deficiency of the male sex hormones. By far the most important of these sex hormones called *androgen*s is testosterone. Testosterone is a molecule that originates in the same sexual organs in men and women but circulates at different amounts. Women have one tenth the testosterone as compared to men but by age forty, their level can be half that of a 20 year-old. In other words women's testosterone goes up as they age and men's goes down. Maybe that's why women live longer.

To learn more about testosterone in the lives of ordinary people, let's eavesdrop on a couple that has been having difficulty. Jane, Russell's wife of several decades, is saying to him, "Russ, you aren't the same any more. After you come home at night all you want to do is sit in front of the TV. You used to like going places and doing things. I'm making an appointment for you to see Dr. Kryger."

"Yes, dear," Russell, a semi-retired stockbroker, concurs. He doesn't have the strength to argue with his wife any more.

Women, like Jane, are often the first to notice these symptoms in their men. In addition to the loss of sexual arousal with weight gain around the waist and loss of strength and agility, their spouse becomes grumpy and distant. Men tend to ignore these symptoms, chalking them up to old age instead of realizing they are not listening to their hormones. Like Jane, it's up to you to keep an eye on your husband's moods and health.

Having scheduled an appointment, Jane and Russell are now sitting in my office. "Russell just isn't the man he used to be," sighs his wife. "He mopes around the house and doesn't seem interested in meeting his clients at work. He used to be the top performer in his division. Now he's just hanging on." She looks around the room. "The worst of it," she says, her voice dropping to a whisper, "is that he doesn't seem to care for me any more. I mean he doesn't even want to have sex." She sighs and fiddles with her purse. "I don't know what's gotten into him."

Russell listens patiently while Jane describes his lack of get-up-and-go. "Russ doesn't play golf on Sundays any more and I can't remember when he went fishing with his buddies. He makes it to work and back but then just sits around. After he goes to bed he tosses and turns and then gets up and makes himself a sandwich. He's gaining weight." She glances at Russell, who nods his head slightly. It takes less effort to go along with his wife's assessment. Then he hears the words that make no sense at all to him.

"You have a classic case of Irritable Male Syndrome." I said, leaning back, waiting for the impact of my words to settle in.

"What?" Russell protests weakly. "I'm always trying to please my wife. There's nothing irritable about me. I do the best I can."

We exchange glances. "I'm sure you do," I said, "but we'll have to do more tests. My hunch is that a small dose of testosterone could help restore your vigor and you'll thank your wife for bringing you in to see me."

During our second visit after reviewing his tests, I write a prescription for testosterone and explain how the testosterone replacement therapy program will work for Russell. He doesn't like the idea, yet knows he'll end up going along with it if he wants to satisfy his wife.

"Why can't my body just regulate itself?" he grumbles. "Isn't hormone replacement unnatural for men?"

After listening to my explanation (which I will give you later), Russell walks out of my office convinced that testosterone will almost certainly be beneficial for him. He feels hopeful and might mention this to his buddies. If he does, which is unlikely, he'll hear some misguided information that may give him second thoughts about hormone therapy. He may be tempted to forget the whole thing.

Like Russell, many men have a hard time accepting that anything is wrong with them especially when they have a mild testosterone deficiency. This is because a hormone deficiency may produce only modest changes at the beginning so a man can be lacking in testosterone or other sex hormones without knowing it. How can you tell your man to ask his doctor to evaluate this important male quality? If your husband or boyfriend is under the age of 45, the loss of morning erections could be the *first sign* that he may have a hormonal deficiency.

Unfortunately most men don't get motivated to do anything about this warning sign until they have lost their ability to have any erections at all! Why do so many men ignore sexual problems when they start noticing them? Here is a sample of some of the reasons.

Many of the effects of low testosterone are troublesome but not serious. The less common effects include an inability to concentrate, diminished interest in daily activities, sleep disturbances, irritability, "grumpy old man syndrome" and depressed moods. This description probably fits a lot of sixty plus men that you know. But it's a big mistake to let your husband's testosterone levels drop so low that he begins experiencing even mild symptoms such as these.

Don't ignore warning signs of a hormonal dysfunction that can be easily corrected if diagnosed early. Men and women need to start being proactive when it comes to their hormone function. It is not normal to lose your mind or memory when you get older. Old age is not associated with feeling grumpy and irritable all the time. Nor is it normal for your joints to become stiff and painful as you age. Are these due entirely to a hormonal shortage?

Two hormones, testosterone and DHEA, jointly regulate the fluid in your joints and keep your tendons and ligaments operating smoothly. Support for this observation comes from studies of youngsters with arthritis who have been found to possess abnormally low levels of testosterone in their joint fluid. Older people with aches and pains in joints and ligaments that improve with exercise may be deficient in testosterone.

Testosterone helps our body rapidly heal the tissues surrounding our joints. Testosterone is also increased in response to moderate exercise, which sort of lubricates our joints. Future studies may show that testosterone deficiency might lead to arthritis and treatment may help improve symptoms of pain and stiffness. In this regard, I am merely making an observation and not advocating an alternative use for testosterone therapy in arthritis.

Let me give you a history of one of my patients. Of course all the names have been changed. Sean, a 72 year-old former concert pianist, shared his experience with low testosterone levels. "Doc, I'm not a saint," Sean said. "I was a big drunk and a drug abuser when I was younger. Now I occasionally eat chocolate, ice cream, pizza, popcorn and other junk. Sometimes I find myself smoking a cigarette or chewing tobacco, but that's rare. I have to tell you what happened."

Sean went on to describe a vigorous exercise program that he now follows, including stretching, weight training and indoor running an hour or more at a time six days a week. But Sean wasn't totally thrilled with his body. He still didn't feel healthy. He knew he needed to lose a few pounds. He also felt that he was not as sharp as he used to be. "I keep forgetting where I left my keys, or daily I lose my glasses," he said. But Sean's greatest loss was his ability to play the piano due to stiffness and aching of his fingers.

Lab tests confirmed that Sean had a testosterone deficiency, so I placed him on a testosterone replacement program using a high potency testosterone cream. We were both pleased to see an improvement in his sense of well-being after only a few weeks. Astoundingly the greatest change was that his ability to play the piano without pain returned after two months of testosterone therapy. He was ecstatic! To this day, Sean practices on the piano more than four hours a day.

Men experiencing problems due to low testosterone levels are often astounded by the benefits of a carefully managed testosterone replacement program. "I can't believe how such a tiny bit of anything could make such a huge difference in my life," Sean told me. "But here I am proof positive. I'm my good-natured, hard-working and hard-playing self again." Sean is very grateful to be playing his beloved piano again.

I am going to say this many times. Testosterone not only strengthens our body and improves our memory but it creates the *essential sense of well-being* that makes us feel alive and motivated, regardless of our age. The value of this capability is immeasurable!

You may wonder, "Can a hormone really make you feel that good and if so, why do men refuse to acknowledge that they need it?" Ego has a lot to do with that, but ignorance of the workings of the male body among men is all too common. That's why it's important to get your spouse to read this book.

As they mature, men should not accept mediocrity as the norm. Vitality, vim and vigor are attainable persist if you have enough testosterone. In your brain, testosterone releases potent endorphins that regulate your perception of pain, creating a state of euphoria, or feeling "high." Spontaneous highs are important for the enjoyment of normal life and the creation of pleasure. There is nothing wrong with feeling naturally high. That's what life is all about.

The Origin of Testosterone and Estrogen

The human body manufactures sex hormones from cholesterol and so we call such related compounds *steroids*. Steroid molecules form a four-ring structure that supports additional side rings furthermore these rings give the molecule its special characteristics. Cholesterol turns out to be the primary substance from which our bodies make testosterone, cortisol, progesterone and estrogen.

The word "steroid" points to the origin of these substances, coming from "sterol" in the word, "cholesterol." The first step in fabricating hormones involves the conversion of cholesterol to pregnenolone. Pregnenolone is not a true hormone, but is the immediate precursor necessary for the synthesis of all steroid hormones. Pregnenolone is found in many places in our bodies, including our adrenals, liver, skin, testicles, ovaries and our brain and the retina at the back of our eyes. Sometimes pregnenolone is called the "grandmother of all hormones" because it is essential for the production of all the sex hormones from cholesterol.

You don't have to go on a high-fat diet to make enough cholesterol. Your body only needs a small amount to assemble your hormones. Unfortunately, cholesterol added to your body from a high animal fat diet contains components such as the oxidized low-density cholesterol (LDL, the bad cholesterol), which can plug up your blood vessels.

But there is something injurious that can happen during this process. The pollutant *dioxin*, discussed in the next chapter, can interfere in the development of *pregnenolone* from cholesterol. Newly incorporated cholesterol cannot always convert to essential hormones because some of the enzymes needed to make the conversion possible are destroyed by dioxin. Unaware of the futility of the task, the liver makes more and more cholesterol, as LDL levels rise higher and higher. Apparently, the cholesterol measure increases in spite of those who claim they don't eat fatty foods.

The amount of cholesterol in our body increases with age even if we don't consume more cholesterol in our diet. One possible explanation is that the pathways that convert cholesterol to the various steroid hormones become impaired as we age. Recognizing the decline in hormones, the body signals its need for more and, as a result, there may be a corresponding increase in cholesterol production by our liver.

This relatively new hypothesis has not been proven but provides intriguing insights. "Hormone restorative therapy," is the term coined by Sergey Dzugan and Arnold Smith, two physicians who undertook to investigate these hormonal deficiencies in aging persons. In a six-year study exploring the factors affecting cholesterol levels, they gave broadly based hormone replacement therapy to the patients in the program. They were not only able to correct their hormone deficiency but restored their cholesterol levels to normal. This amazing response occurred in every one of their patients!

Cholesterol levels have jumped to incredible highs with the advent of fast foods and "meat on every table." We need more research about toxic exposure from animal fat. Then we will understand why the accumulation of environmental toxins over time could increase our cholesterol counts while decreasing our hormones.

Hormones Are Not Sexist—Why Don't Men Ask for Help?

As we review the endocrine system and the neurosteroids, you will start to realize that testosterone acts much like a neurohormone. In the brain, testosterone can convert to estrogen, creating new brain cells or neurons. DHT or dihydrotestosterone, converted in your brain from testosterone, is responsible for your human sexual drive. When testosterone enhances libido and energy in women, it peaks just before ovulation. In men, testosterone amplifies strength and decreases body fat. Testosterone boosts energy, memory, improves libido and sexual performance. In other words, testosterone is a very versatile hormone. It can convert to estrogen or DHT and as a rule; the estrogen produced by men and women comes from testosterone.

Although men make greater amounts of testosterone than women, the hormone is essential for all human beings. As a matter of fact though the same hormones are present in both sexes for we are the same species, sometimes, owing to the marked differences between us, we wonder about that.

Whenever I speak to women about the men in their lives they ask me why men don't ask for help when they are having trouble with heart problems, diabetes, or depression. All of them want to know how they can help their men make positive changes. I often respond as follows:

Testosterone helps your man to deal with novel situations, challenges and find solutions to problems. Many men are not aware they have a shortage of testosterone as they lose their capacity to find life interesting and challenging. They feel as if they are useless, old and washed up. They have lost their motivation. Without testosterone flowing through their veins, men feel less masculine, less secure and less interested in anything, including sex. Testosterone deficiency is more common than we once thought.

Testosterone is the undisputed king of the hormones. As a steroid hormone directed to perform vital tasks in regulating, stimulating and controlling our bodies and our brains, testosterone has the potential for helping men and women alike to experience sexual, physical and emotional pleasure. Are you ready for this; it might help you do a better job in your career. No, I'm not talking about a macho approach in the boardroom. Simply put, testosterone is a hormone that is vital for making decisions.

Boosting strength, promoting the building of muscles and speeding up the healing process after an injury are common effects, but remember too that testosterone encourages risk-taking, which can be an advantage in business. As many of you know, success in life is often dependent on your willingness to take chances, to experiment, to follow your instincts and not be discouraged by the mistakes of others who did not know what they were doing or how to handle difficult situations.

Low testosterone has powerful effects on the human brain. As testosterone falls below vital levels, men and women suffer a loss of memory, difficulty orienting in space, i.e., bumping into things, on top of lagging sexual desire. The negative effects of low testosterone include sluggishness and a loss of strength and endurance.

Consideration of hormonal deficiency is a critical part of the medical evaluation of any patient with sexual dysfunction, memory problems or low libido. Lately studies have confirmed that testosterone may help prevent Alzheimer's dementia and is essential for normal human brain function. Based on a considerable amount of scientific data, we now believe that early on testosterone modifies brain structures, particularly the *hippocampus*, that part of the brain that is responsible for memory in humans.

From birth until about age 21, men enjoy heightened levels of testosterone. Usually reaching a peak from puberty to young adulthood, testosterone then declines throughout the rest of their life. The amount of testosterone in our body is carefully regulated by an intricate system of checks and balances. The testosterone-regulating hormone, dubbed luteinizing hormone (LH), registers if there is too much testosterone and stimulates the production of this sex hormone until we have just the right balance. *This self-regulation takes place in both sexes.*

In response to our biologic clock, our hormones rise and fall depending on the time of day. Typically, the highest testosterone count in men under age 40 occurs during the early waking hours from 6 to 8 a.m. By early morning, a man's internal clock has signaled his body to make more testosterone until it reaches its maximum level generating a firm morning erection. The onset of daylight makes testosterone decrease only to build up again during the night.

These daily peaks and valleys or hormone fluctuations become less pronounced as you age. The most important form of testosterone is labeled the free testosterone and it is equal to only two to four percent of the total testosterone. This may seem like a small portion but this type of testosterone creates all the hormonal outcomes in the human body.

Regrettably, few men or women bother to find out what their normal testosterone levels are *before* they have a problem. Even if a person knows how much testosterone is circulating in their body, *optimal* levels vary so widely from one man or women to another that accurate treatment to adjust these levels is tricky but not impossible.

Proper hormonal balancing requires both experience and sensitivity on the part of the physician. Yet normal ranges are all we have to deal with. Both laboratory tests and clinical presentation are essential for proper diagnosis. Interested physicians should monitor research in the field. Two comprehensive papers published in 2005, at long last present medical doctors with age-specific normal ranges for DHEA, free and total testosterone and androstenedione.(See Appendix B).

Consider the three primary sex hormones: testosterone, estrogen and progesterone as the heritage of the entire human species rather than favoring one sex or the other. For instance, testosterone intensifies that all-important sense of well-being for all human beings and both sexes respond to testosterone supplements with increased muscular growth and sexual desire. Hormones have built-in safety factors and every hormone has an opposing regulator. Progesterone may be central in balancing the negative effects of testosterone or estrogen when it acts as a hormone regulator or neurohormone.

What Does Testosterone Do for Women?

While women have about one tenth the amount of testosterone found in men, this hormone plays a vital role in a woman's "ability to be aroused... and in her appetite for being sexual," according to Dr. Rosemary Basson, with the Center for Sexuality, Gender Identity and Reproductive Health in British Columbia. Dr. Basson points out that testosterone plays significant roles in women. These include promoting bone growth, increasing bone density, stimulating the production of red blood cells, promoting muscular development, plus improving moods and sex drive. Testosterone may also lower total cholesterol and LDL and decrease insulin resistance.

A woman with high testosterone is the owner of a firm body with a flat abdomen and high energy. She can be sexually aggressive and especially attractive but not at all masculine. Testosterone (T) nurtures sexual desire and heightens a woman's sensitivity to sexual stimulation. The result is a deeper sense of physical gratification during sexual intercourse. These subtle feelings are missing in women with low T levels.

The first indication that a woman may have a low T level is usually a lack of sexual desire and erotic thoughts or dreams. An article concerning women who were deficient in testosterone appeared in the February 2005 issue of *Endocrine News*. The main point made by Dr. Glenn Braunstein, of the UCLA School of Medicine, was that women have been receiving various types of testosterone supplementation to treat the loss of sexual responsiveness for over 50 years, yet its effectiveness for libido has never been properly investigated.

Currently there are no FDA-approved testosterone treatments for women. Nonetheless, testosterone has been used clinically in women for decades. Any woman with a loss of sexual desire due to removal of her ovaries (the major production center of testosterone) feels remarkably better when testosterone is replaced. This is called an "anecdotal response" implying it has not been adequately tested.

Subsequently, most women have been forced to use T products made for men. The irony is that the testosterone products marketed for a man are strong enough for a woman when used in tiny doses. At this point in time, many men do not use the same products made for them, while women are deprived of the matching therapy.

Again, it is interesting to note that inclusive of the year 2005, no products exist for testosterone therapy for women. What is the reason? Over the past three years, Susan Davis, an expert in female hormone therapy, has successfully tested Intrinsa®, a transdermal T patch for women on hundreds of women in Melbourne, Australia. Late in 2004, a panel of advisers, from a competing pharmaceutical company, BioSante, told the FDA that in light of the possible risks for heart disease and stroke, more research was needed before Intrinsa® should be approved. Another few years of research were suggested as the FDA went along with them.

Just as it does in men, testosterone therapy helps to heighten sexual desire in women. Women derive half of their testosterone from their ovaries and half from their adrenal glands. Their T levels peak between the age of 20 and 30, diminish by about 50 percent after menopause, but never disappear completely. It is interesting to note that some postmenopausal women may even notice an increase in testosterone as they age.

Menopause should not be considered a disease but an accepted transition in women from fertility to cessation of menstruation. Many women find menopause to be a positive experience since they no longer have to worry about pregnancy and can enjoy luxurious sex in the morning without interruption from children or carpools.

Weight gain is common but is not a part of the menopause. As Dr. Patricia Allen, author of *Staying Married... and Loving It,* stated on a recent TV interview *Embracing menopause,* "Hormones do not make you fat, it is what you eat that makes you fat." This is true but difficult for many people to accept. However, many postmenopausal women complain of vaginal dryness along with a decreased desire to exercise, which could contribute to weight gain after menopause.

Women with low T levels can suffer from symptoms that are similar to those experienced by men, including lowered libido and decreased ability to achieve sexual arousal, plus fatigue and negative moods. Studies examining testosterone replacement therapy (TRT) in women have been few; as a consequence further study is clearly necessary to establish the validity of TRT in women.

Eventually age drives most women's testosterone down as it does in men. As their testosterone levels drop, previously youthful women begin aging rapidly, often becoming overweight and more passive. Women with low testosterone develop heart disease sooner and lose their memory faster than women with normal levels. Side effects are rare though there is a slight risk of masculinizing side effects such as acne, facial hair and a lowered voice in women who take *too much* testosterone.

In addition to aging, other causes for the dwindling of women's androgen levels include the use of birth control pills, the process of pregnancy and breast feeding and the use of a popular class of anti-depressants named specific serotonin re-uptake inhibitors or SSRIs. Prozac®, Paxil®, Zoloft® and Lexapro® are four common SSRIs that have been shown to cause a decreased libido, as well as an inability to reach orgasm. As you may know, a delayed orgasm is not always negative for women, but men suffer great frustration when orgasm fails to occur at the optimal moment.

While many of the same hormones function on an equal opportunity basis in both men and women, the truth is that when it comes to sex a woman doesn't think like a man. She doesn't see men the same way that men see women.

While many men equate love with sex "If you loved me you would have sex with me", women need love to feel sexy. "Do you love me? Just tell me you love me," is a woman's constant plea. A woman's craving for love starts the trickle of hormones flowing to provide adequate vaginal lubrication. Women generally perceive sexual craving as "love." It develops only after multiple orgasms and a feeling of trust in her partner. From the woman's perspective, the bond that forms can last a lifetime.

Keep in mind that men's feelings are quite different from women. Men's cycles of sex or love have no set pattern. "Good sex leads to love," is a philosophy often quoted by many men. I've learned from patients that in many cases while a man sees woman as the perpetuator of the human race, he is more interested in a woman's physical attributes than in the woman's deep-seated emotions. This may be why many men are able to enjoy sex with several women, once aroused by the energy of their hormones.

A woman, on the other hand, needs more than hormones to enjoy sex. She must be extremely interested in the man and feel he cares for her on an emotional level, not just for her body. Today, fulfilling sex and loving are equally hard to find. In spite of everything, if you are married, love is a lot more complicated than just having sex or getting aroused. A hormonal imbalance can lead to a mismatch, fostering a faltering relationship. Sensing this, many women, eager to save their relationships, seek professional counsel. Unfortunately they can't solve the crisis themselves. They must have the cooperation of their partner to save their relationship.

Strong arguments regarding the use of testosterone replacement therapy or TRT in women have been made from both sides. Some say that TRT is generally inappropriate for women and that sexual issues are better dealt with through counseling, psychotherapy, stress reduction and other psychosocial approaches. In contrast, treating symptoms that are clearly linked to low levels of free or circulating testosterone can significantly improve quality of life according to medical experts in the field: Jennifer Berman, Susan Davis and Jeanne Alexander.

The practical obstacles to precise testosterone supplementation in women are significant. This is partly for physiologic reasons; where men make testosterone in the testes, testosterone production in women is divided between the adrenal glands and the ovaries. The precursor hormones, DHEA and androstenedione, convert into about half the required female testosterone. In some women, particularly as they grow older, these conversions do not occur and they may end up running low in testosterone. Other women have plenty of testosterone as they age. This information may lead you to wonder if couples lose their hormone levels all at once, losing interest in sex after menopause.

For women experiencing menopause, the male hormones inevitably decline. Another researcher, Dr. Lorraine Dennerstein, also from Melbourne, concluded from her studies that the primary drivers for a woman's libido are androgens. Less than a milligram a day of a testosterone supplement, seems to improve sexual health in testosterone deficient women without bringing on any masculine traits. Menopausal women appear to benefit from testosterone with increased energy and an improved sense of well-being.

Women Have More Oxytocin Than Men

While women may have less testosterone, when it comes to certain other hormones, they surpass men. Oxytocin is such a hormone. Two young graduate students, Cindy Meston and Penny Frohlich, found evidence that oxytocin and vasopressin, another hormone we will discuss later, have an additive effect on sexual function. Their thesis reports that in both sexes circulating levels of oxytocin increase during sexual arousal and orgasm.

According to Dr. George Gimpl at Guttenberg University in Germany, the action of oxytocin on the central nervous system includes creating and directing complex activities involved in reproduction and the care of infants. For instance, oxytocin exerts potent anti-stress effects that facilitate the bonding of males to females and encourages mothering and fathering behaviors. The stress-reducing effect of oxytocin promotes a positive connection between mother and child and father and child. Oxytocin effects on maternal behavior help mothers nurture their offspring and intensify the bonding needed to keep a father in the family unit.

Oxytocin has cast a magic spell on lovers throughout the centuries. The bewildering, seductive powers of oxytocin continue to guide us through the stages of arousal and orgasm. If you've ever been in love, you've experienced the power of oxytocin. Just touching a woman's skin releases oxytocin, instilling a desire to be caressed and loved.

Oxytocin depends in part, on estrogen to perform. Because women have far more estrogen than men, the arousal effect of touching is intensified in women. In addition to increasing a woman's sexual desire, oxytocin prepares her body for intercourse by increasing vaginal lubrication. Women, who are capable of experiencing more intense orgasms, generally have higher levels of oxytocin in their systems. If orgasms and ejaculations increase, that makes oxytocin sound like a great hormone. But there's more!

The presence of oxytocin reinforces *monogamy*—the desire for a single sexual partner. One researcher found that the brains of animals that mate with a single member of their species have higher concentrations of oxytocin than do animals with many sexual partners. In every animal species, oxytocin regulates birthing and nursing behaviors. From love to birth to the production of milk, oxytocin rules!

When sufficient oxytocin is present, sexual posturing increases as courtship and couple bonding is strengthened. Since higher oxytocin levels correspond to more intense orgasmic contractions in men and women, someday we may be able to buy sexual bonding and commitment in a spray bottle. A nasal spray derived from oxytocin to induce sexual arousal is already in clinical trials. In the meantime, listen carefully to the needs of your sexual partners who may be searching for that spark to revitalize their own passion.

Are Men and Women Mismatched Sexually?

As a consequence of our circadian rhythms, a man's sexual interest peaks in the morning because that's when hormones are at their crest. For practical reasons, this is not always an ideal time to take pleasure in making love. The day is just beginning and the kids have to get off to school. We all have to go to work on time or keep appointments and so on. Late evening is far more convenient for sexual activity creating an ideal niche in the daily schedule. It's quiet. We are comfortably full. The bed is soft and inviting. The kids are in bed and it's dark. This seems like the best time to snuggle and enjoy a taste of blissful sex. But is it really?

"Honey," John, a local fireman, says as he pulls off his socks and climbs between the sheets. "That was a lovely meal, but I'm stuffed."

"You're right" Linda, his lovely, wife of 15 years, murmurs, turning towards him. "It was delicious. I loved the crème caramel dessert."

"You know," John, continues, "I had a lousy day at work. I'd like to just settle in for a refreshing sleep. How about you?"

"Sure," Linda exhales with an unromantic sigh, turning off the light.

Two nights later, John has a renewed enthusiasm for sex. Comfortable and not satiated with a big meal, he pulls Linda to his side giving her a big hug. Hand on her back he guides her toward the bed. She kisses him, knowing what's coming; she playfully struggles to free herself from his embrace. "Not tonight, John," she whispers. "I have a headache. I really do." Sound familiar?

Couples like this are insensitive to their sexual rhythms and as a result may become deeply frustrated. Because they are not in tune with their hormones, when one partner doesn't feel in the mood, cuddling or kissing can create arousal and satisfy the other partner. It's worth a try since this behavior essentially raises testosterone.

When diminished hormone levels return to normal, most people feel good. Linda and John are just two of the millions of couples who need to pay attention to their hormone levels and normal cycles. They will each come out winners when they work out a pattern of sexual fulfillment that is mutually satisfactory.

As mentioned earlier, women are different from men when it comes to sex. Whether her desire for sex begins in her head or in her heart, the reality is that a woman needs enough testosterone in order to feel sexually drawn to her partner. That same partner needs an adequate amount to respond equally. Our brain can be thought of as our most important sex organ because that's where sexual arousal begins. It is in the brain that testosterone becomes either DHT or estrogen. The direction this conversion takes will determine whether our sex drive is adequate.

How can you use this information? Well, here are some strategies to help you to reach your own level of optimal sexual performance.

First of all and most important, avoid tobacco in any form. Smoking cigarettes is the *number one* cause of impotence in men (and women). Limit alcohol intake, for this is the second most common cause of sexual difficulty. Delay sexual activity until more than two hours after drinking alcohol or eating.

Second: Plan sexual activity for a time when your energy and hormone level are the highest and you are rested and relaxed. Yes, morning is better than evening. In the early morning a man's gets more easily provoked. Experiment with different sexual positions to find what is most comfortable for you and your partner.

Third: Maximize the use of nonsexual intimate touching and enhance sexual expression through the use of your senses. This is what I mean when I say the brain is a powerful sexual organ; it encompasses all our senses. Fantasy is a powerful sexual tool.

There is nothing wrong with self-stimulation when needed to reduce anxiety, help with sleep or provide general pleasure. Using self-help books that cover the subject of sexual activity is practical and intelligent. Incorporating Masters and Johnson's *sensate focus* helps couples learn what each partner likes or dislikes and vice versa.

You may assume from these ideas, that the loss of your sex drive is simply related to your attitude and you can handle these concerns on your own. That may be true for some but it's always best if you talk to your doctor about your low sexual energy and ask him if your condition can be treated with hormone supplements. Do not hesitate to follow your doctor's recommendation to restore normal sexual function. Hormones are safe and effective even in minuscule doses.

Specific hormones are essential for normal sexual function. Whatever your age, you should retain a desire for sexual activity on some level until the end. If you are a man you should have enough testos-terone to achieve and maintain an erection for your partner's sexual pleasure throughout your life. If you are a woman, you should pos-sess enough oxytocin to give you the ability to enjoy arousal, intimate contact and orgasm with your partner at any age.

2

OUR JUMBLED HORMONES

How Do Our Genes Work?

Genes regulate our hormones and hormones in turn affect genes. An incredibly complex set of commands and interactions known as the genetic code governs our genes and makes life possible, healthy and satisfying. Each of us possesses an estimated 66,000 genes, the architects of the human body. Our genes set our hormones in motion and hormones, in turn, drive our emotions, our sexual responses, our height and weight, the length of our lives and many other character-istics. When things go wrong, our hormones immediately coordinate their powers to combat the challenge. Usually they win.

Jumbled hormones can scramble our genes. As remarkable as our ability to recover from disease and injury may be, it is nevertheless true that a flaw or injury to one strand of our genetic structure can have repercussions for a lifetime and into future generations. It has now been proven that our grandmother's genes can affect our life and that of our children. Grandmothers who smoked cigarettes while pregnant can increase the incidence of asthma in their grandchildren, even if the mothers themselves do not smoke. Sometimes our hormones become entangled for other reasons and sometimes our genes fail to produce essential proteins. Genetic tests are now available to detect some of the defects in hormonal regulation.

Can We Get Cancer from Estrogen?

If you read the paper today or watch the news, you know that hormone replacement therapy (HRT) is not risk-free. Most women, who call or visit me about the health problems of the men in their lives, are concerned about hormonal side effects. Visit any bookstore, library or website and you'll find an enormous amount of information on HRT for women. Because new studies have suggested that some of these treatments are dangerous, women frequently begin conversations with me by reviewing recent medical information they have found online. Before exploring possible treatment for their companions, they want to know if *any* hormone replacement program is a good idea.

Their concern is reasonable. Typically, women worried about their own safety, will ask if I believe estrogen replacement therapy is good or bad. There are no quick answers to this question. But the latest studies reveal why it's critical for women and men to be up to date on this vital medical issue. While this book is primarily directed at men's health, let's look specifically at the related woman's perspective.

On January 1, 2001, the National Institute of Environmental Health added estrogen to the list of chemicals known to *cause cancer*. The ominous news came after studies showed that women who take estrogen supplements to cope with their menopause have a stronger risk of uterine cancer, heart disease, dementia and breast or uterine cancer than those who did not use estrogen.

Current evidence indicates that many tumors, especially in the breast and the prostate, feed on estrogen. The exact mechanism that causes tumor growth is not fully understood, but we do know that a specific enzyme, aromatase, helps create estrogen from testosterone and that estrogen, in turn, stimulates the multiplication of all cells. Yet it's not all bad since estrogen can make brain cells proliferate as easily as breast cells.

Estrogen is present in men and women but excess estrogen can cause sexual dysfunction, prostate cancer and breast cancer. Breast cancer was reported in three transgender males who underwent sex-change surgery to become females and received prolonged treatment with estrogen. Primary breast cancer occasionally develops in the breasts of men with prostate cancer who are treated with estrogen to suppress testosterone.

Pharmaceutical companies are therefore jumping on the anti-estrogen bandwagon by developing estrogen blockers like Novaldex or Tamoxifen and Arimidex or Anastrozole to treat breast cancer and preventing a recurrence. These anti-estrogens have proven most effective over the long run in saving the lives of women with breast cancer. They are also useful in raising the degree of testosterone in elderly men with low levels. Other drugs that interfere with the cancer-inducing properties of estrogen are also being developed and not a minute too soon, because currently some 60 to 75 percent of all breast cancers are *estrogen dependent*.

Don't men need estrogen? Yes, they do. Estrogen plays an important role in a man's testicular development and is a central hormone for both men and women. But high levels of estrogen can also have serious negative effects in men, including testicular cancer, undescended testicles, low sperm counts, shrinking sex organs and the inevitable sexual dysfunction. Our concern is not for the estrogen our body turns out biologically but the estrogen that is foreign to unprotected human tissues.

Let me clarify. All hormones manufactured by your body are self-regulating. Hormones that come from outside your body, or synthetic hormones, are not regulated by this built-in system and can mix-up your endocrine system with disastrous results. In fact many of the problems endocrinologists treat every day are the result of contamination by synthetic hormones. The good news is that men can reverse this damage with the help of their personal physician. Again, let me emphasize that this is not a do-it-yourself project. You must seek treatment from a qualified health care professional.

A Primer On Estrogen For Men

While this book focuses on men, it's vital to understand estrogen, the hormone responsible for the creation of the female body. Many new patients are surprised to learn that hormones present in our environment can jumble the endocrine system quite easily. We call these estrogen-like compounds environmental estrogens or *xenoestrogens*. We are talking about all-pervading toxic substances like dioxin and organic polychlorides, abbreviated as TCDD, PVCs or PCBs. These mimic the chemical activity of estrogen in the human body.

For years these compounds have been shrugged off as not powerful enough to cause serious problems. Unfortunately the problem with the dioxin-type estrogen mimics is that differences in their structure cannot be regulated by the body's hormone feedback systems. In other words, we have no safety net when it comes to exposure to these toxic compounds.

Though estrogen formed outside the human body is a proven carcinogen, medical researchers have agreed that the benefits of estrogen therapy for women far outweigh the risks. Estrogen therapy for women with a deficiency and hot flashes or osteoporosis continues despite evidence that estrogen supplements could be responsible for increased cancer of all sexual organs.

Estradiol (E2) is the form of estrogen that has been linked most directly to a higher risk of cancer in the breast and prostate. This variety of estrogen is considered bioidentical to the human 17-beta estradiol. E2 is the active ingredient in FDA-approved female hormone supplements including patches, pills, creams and vaginal rings.

This is not to say that a "safe estrogen level" cannot be the goal. More on these products is found in the appendix.

The good news about estrogen therapy is that estradiol is responsible for increasing cerebral blood flow, stimulating brain cells and the speed at which messages cross the gap between nerves—the "synapse." For this reason women appear smarter than men as long as they have enough estrogen.

Today doctors can protect women against some of the negative effects of estradiol or E2, by adding progesterone or testosterone to their hormone replacement therapy program. The addition of these hormones to the mix can also cancel the higher risk of breast and uterine cancer associated with "unopposed" estrogen therapy. Unopposed estrogen therapy refers to the use of E2 alone for the treatment of menopause.

You may have heard that estrogen supplements reduce the risk of age-related senility or heart attacks, but evidence was lacking and the long-term studies were not performed. We do know from recent research that there is a hormone that protects men's and women's hearts, but it is testosterone, not estradiol. In clinical trials, appropriate levels of the *male* hormone, testosterone, reduced the risk of heart disease, Alzheimer's and age-related senility among men *and* women. As men mature, the balance between testosterone and estradiol may tilt in favor of E2 production.

It is easy to assume that for women, estrogen is more important than testosterone. This assumption is not totally accurate. Androstenedione, a testosterone precursor, is more important for women than it is for men. This hormone can directly become estrone, the primary estrogen, which has regulatory powers over female reproduction as well as male sperm formation.

Androstenedione, notorious in bodybuilding circles as *andro*, is able to bypass conversion to estrone, the final stage of estrogen metabolism and become testosterone instead. Numerous studies suggest that androstenedione—once sold over the counter for athletes—converts to estrogen rather than more testosterone as preferred by men.

Consequently, young boys who are looking for muscles may end up with breasts.

When estrogen levels increase beyond acceptable limits, the ratio of testosterone to estrogen is tipped. Changes in the interrelationship of these hormones stimulate the growth and transformation of malignant cells. This is a dangerous situation with serious consequences ranging from cancer to a heightened risk of certain autoimmune diseases in which the body attacks its own tissues. The production of higher than normal E2 levels in either sex can lead to the formation of blood clots, unwanted breast development, heart attacks, along with depression, aggression, moodiness and violent tempers.

For more than three decades, doctors have debated whether estrogen replacement therapy (ERT) using estradiol alone was more effective than full hormone replacement therapy (HRT) including testosterone and progesterone. While the silly battle of acronyms rages on—ERT versus HRT or TRT versus bioidentical hormone replacement therapy or BHRT—pharmaceutical companies rigorously promote horse-based estrogens as the standard of care. The hormone Premarin®, probably the most popular of these estrogens, was derived from pregnant mare's urine (PREgnant MAre's urINe).

Horse urine may soon be replaced by newer hormone medications, a bioidentical estrogen or progesterone, which is more natural. These products will be on the market soon and a few are already available to pharmacists at a low cost for compounding into gels and creams, according to doctors' prescriptions.

Why would doctors prescribe synthetic estrogens for women when real estrogens are available? The answer is both financial and promotional. First of all, hormones that occur in nature can be toxic and second of all, no man-made hormones are really genuine. The perception has been that Premarin has been used for so long that it must be safe and effective. This same reasoning was also used by the pharmaceutical company Merck, which made Vioxx® and the combination E2-T pill, known as Estratest® (by Solvay) for women.

Estratest was placed on the market without FDA approval almost two decades ago. It contained methyltestosterone as the primary form of testosterone along with estradiol. In small doses this synthetic hormone seemed safe but long-term studies were not carried out, other than for controlling hot flashes. Estratest is the only combination estrogen-testosterone product currently on the market. Out of interest, all hormones used in FDA-approved products are synthesized to resemble the identical hormone in the body.

After more than 50 years of use and many studies, evidence is still inconsistent about any relationship between the use of HRT and the risk of breast cancer. The absence of convincing evidence is reassuring because it implies that any risk of breast cancer from hormone replacement therapy is minimal. HRT use lasting less than five years seems to confer no increased risk of breast cancer. By contrast, women using HRT for 10 to 15 years seem to have a minimal but slightly higher risk of breast cancer. Again, these risks are insignificant in comparison to the beneficial effects.

Is Synthetic Progesterone More Dangerous Than Synthetic Estrogen?

For the past 25 years it was assumed that women had the benefits of life-enhancing hormone treatments that were both safe and effective. It was assumed that this is why they outlived men. New research from the Women's Health Initiative (WHI) put traditional hormone replacement therapy in a bad light. After long-term studies lasting over a quarter of a century and involving thousands of women, news reports indicated that equine (horse) estrogens and synthetic progestins did *not* protect women against heart disease but actually increased their risk of breast cancer and heart attacks if they smoked.

Provera® (medroxyprogesterone), man-made progesterone, has been blamed for breast cancer and the variety of side effects seen with hormone replacement therapy. Provera can cause depression, irritability

41

and sleep deprivation. The progestins seem to create a greater risk as compared to horse estrogens, which can act just like human estrogens. Since companies can't obtain a patent for biologic hormones, there was no competitive advantage in marketing them to women. As a result, pharmaceuticals focused on substituting synthetic hormones that could be patent-protected for up to 20 years.

Women around the world have been using the potentially dangerous synthetic hormones Premarin® and Provera® (recently combined as Prempro® by Wyeth) for menopausal symptoms for almost three decades. This is unfortunate, since some women can get the same relief by using safe and biological menopause treatment with bioidentical hormones rather than synthetic hormones.

Again, I have to stress that *all* hormones are synthesized in the lab to act as either bioidentical compounds or metabolic byproducts of hormones. Synthetic hormones, as described in this book, refer to those hormones which are NOT the same as the physical hormones produced by endocrine glands. Calling hormones *natural* refers to the bioidentical hormones as mentioned by Suzanne Somers in her book, *The Sexy Years*.

An article in Endocrine News, July 2005, written by endocrinologists, Leslie Salomone and Richard Santen from the University of Virginia, was titled *Bioidentical Hormone Replacement: Myths and Facts*. In commenting on Ms. Somers statements these two doctors agreed with the following facts:

1. Women should be encouraged to discuss bioidentical hormones replacement therapy (BRHT) and voice questions or concerns about the menopause with their medical providers.

2. Tailoring of therapy to the individual patient is appropriate.

3. The "one-pill-fits-all approach" is *not* the best way to manage menopause.

4. Bioidentical hormones are synthesized in the laboratory and are "natural" compounds—exact replicas of the hormones created by a woman's ovaries.

5. Monitoring of blood levels of administered estradiol is beneficial to the patients who are *not* responding well to therapy.

They disagreed with her comments regarding weight gain with menopause and stated that her all-inclusive claims that BHRT is a *solution* to "controlling weight, avoiding diseases of aging and restoring energy, vitality, a youthful glow, sexuality, a slim figure, a good attitude, healthier bones, a healthier heart and a healthier brain," are only partially correct. Their position gives considerable credence to the use of BHRT in the treatment of postmenopausal women.

Bioidentical estrogens benefit a woman's intelligence through neuroprotective effects while stimulating neuron growth in the brain. These effects give rise to increased verbal fluency and protection against the decline in memory or reaction time that commonly occurs with aging.

The Effects of Bioidentical Progesterone in Women

To put this hormone in proper perspective, let's review the role of *true progesterone* in women. When cells in a woman's ovary make progesterone during the monthly release of the egg, they prepare the lining of the uterus to absorb and protect the fertilized egg. This activity takes place in the uterus but a woman also needs a good supply of progesterone in order to become fertile. Often dubbed the "pregnancy hormone," progesterone is known for its role in protecting the health of a pregnant woman. To carry out its helpful role, progesterone skyrockets during pregnancy to a *thousand times* normal levels.

The body rapidly absorbs biological progesterone taken by mouth. By the time it reaches the liver, most of it is no longer active so few benefits are received. To deal with this problem, researchers developed synthetic progesterone products that are not absorbed as rapidly and thus assure the delivery of adequate progesterone.

As I've explained, hormones are intricately connected. Changes in the concentration of one hormone, affect the amounts of other hormones. In men, for example, a deficiency in either testosterone or progesterone can create a deficiency in hormones such as estrogen or DHEA and vice versa.

Males and females normally secrete one to five milligrams of progesterone daily. About ten days before menstruation, this level rises during the egg-releasing stage of the menstrual cycle. This monthly cycle repeats itself if the egg is not fertilized or implanted into the uterus. Progesterone levels rise and then fall just before bleeding signals the start of a woman's menstrual cycle. This premenstrual time is termed the *progesterone withdrawal phase*. For some women it is an extremely anxious, nervous time. A number of women report symptoms of depression: crying easily, feeling low self-esteem and losing interest in their close female friends. The premenstrual signs signal women that their period is coming.

Other problems during the premenstrual time of the month range from mild to severe cramps and wild emotional swings that can drive women to violence. The well-publicized premenstrual syndrome, or PMS, has been used as a defense for murder in the UK. Fortunately, not all women suffer PMS to such a degree. In its milder forms, PMS is quite benign with cramping and irritability. PMS is common in women with irregular menstrual cycles, little exercise, endometriosis or a family history of miscarriages.

In his book, *Natural Progesterone*, Dr. John Lee wrote, "Women whose doctors are giving them excessive supplemental estrogen, a different problem must be faced. Excessive estrogen in circumstances of deficient progesterone induces a decrease in receptor sensitivity. An important function of progesterone is to restore the normal sensitivity of estrogen receptors. When progesterone is restored, estrogen receptor sensitivity is also restored. It is not surprising that, in these cases, some women develop symptoms of estrogen dominance: water retention, headaches, weight gain, and swollen breasts, when progesterone is first supplemented. Obviously, the estrogen dose must be lowered. If this is done too rapidly, however, hot flushes can occur.

The key is to reduce estrogen gradually while progesterone is being restored."

Bioidentical progesterone acts to reduce both estrogens and androgens in the brain and it can down-regulate the estrogen receptors. This means that progesterone blocks these receptors that can make women irritable, leading to a beneficial calming effect, allowing them to have a restful sleep. Progesterone has other benefits, too.

Doctors today have several options in treating women with hormonal replacement therapy. Bioidentical estrogens are currently available in transdermal patches, vaginal rings and oral tablets. Solvay has just released a new gel form of estrogen, EstroGel®. Two bioidentical progesterones are available as Prometrium® from Solvay and Prochieve® from Columbia Laboratories. Holistic therapies and phytoestrogens are now competing for the estrogen market while there are over a dozen estrogen products approved by the FDA.

Remembering the Mother of All Hormones

Progesterone is one of several female sex hormones known as *progestins*. The most important progestin, progesterone, is made from cholesterol in the ovaries, testicles and in the adrenal glands. When the body breaks down progesterone, it becomes either testosterone or estrogen. The metabolic breakdown of progesterone also contributes to the production of many other hormones we will discuss throughout this book, including cortisol, aldosterone, estradiol and DHEA in addition to testosterone. This is why progesterone can be thought of as the "mother of all hormones."

I call progesterone the "forgotten hormone" because it is hardly ever considered in male hormone replacement therapy. Progesterone can be made from the conversion of cholesterol to pregnenolone in the adrenal gland and it can also be produced in the brain. Progesterone in the brain is able to mimic many of the actions of specific neurotransmitters that regulate sleep, moods, appetite and deep sleep breathing. Because of these numerous capabilities, progesterone is considered a neurosteroid when it is produced in the brain. This may explain some of its effectiveness in PMS.

The role of progesterone in men is not well understood but the amount of progesterone produced by men is identical to that of women. There is data and a growing body of literature indicating that progesterone not only influences sexual behavior in males, but also does so in diverse vertebrate species. Given that it appears to be capable of inducing either male-typical or female-typical sexual behavior in various species, more studies are needed.

According to John Lee, MD, achieving balance is the key when it comes to progesterone supplementation. He states, "The goal is to restore normal physiologic levels of bioavailable progesterone. Progesterone/estrogen balance is the key … In PMS, for example, stress is often a factor. Stress increases cortisol production. Cortisol blockades some progesterone receptors and thereby inhibits progesterone function. To compete with this cortisol blockade, topical progesterone in the range of 30 to 40 mg/day is initially required to achieve a beneficial effect."

Today there are about six different brands of synthetic progestins on the market but there are only two bioidentical FDA-approved progesterones, Procheive® and Prometrium®. Next to estrogen, progestins are the second most common hormone prescribed for women. You have probably heard of Provera®, synthetic progesterone manufactured by Wyeth. Women complain of increased breast tenderness, bloating of the abdomen and ever-changing moods when progestins such as Provera are used premenstrually. These symptoms are almost identical to those of patients with a deficiency of progesterone.

I do not recommend the use of synthetic progesterone, which lasts all day, because too much progesterone can be harmful. An excess of this hormone in the body can create unusual symptoms by competing with another hormone known as aldosterone, the salt-regulating hormone. Aldosterone comes from the adrenal gland and affects the functioning of the kidney. Too much progesterone from small amounts of synthetic progestins can stop the kidneys from excreting salt, leading to fluid retention and swollen ankles. When men or women crave salt, it is usually because their body levels of salt are low. An oversupply of progesterone could be another reason. Symptoms, including cravings for salt and sugar, may be triggered by excessive progesterone. But, like most hormones, there is a good and bad side to progesterone.

Progesterone supplements can halt premenstrual cravings for sweets in women who experience enormous drops in their progesterone levels before their period starts. Taking progesterone in small doses of 10 to 100 milligrams a day safely boosts low premenstrual levels into the normal range. In recent times, progesterone has been added to estrogen replacement therapy for its beneficial role in reducing the cancer-causing action of estradiol on the breast and uterus. Women with a uterus can therefore benefit when progesterone is added to HRT, canceling some of the negative effects of unopposed estrogen.

Treatment with progesterone may even help protect men against prostate cancer. Progesterone affects our rate and depth of breathing. Olympic athletes from China have already turned to progesterone supplements to improve their breathing while running. The benefit came from the fact that progesterone reduces carbon dioxide levels in the blood and lungs. Next time you huff and puff when walking up a hill, consider the fact that a progesterone deficiency might be causing your shortness of breath.

The ability of progesterone to stimulate breathing has been known for years, According to Meir Kryger, a Canadian physician and a national sleep expert, this hormone protects pregnant women and young women from disordered breathing and snoring during sleep. Progesterone, in its role as a neurohormone, acts as a tranquilizer in the brain. You may have heard that some people stop breathing temporarily while sleeping. About nine percent of adult women and

24 percent of adult men have this condition called *obstructive sleep apnea.*

My patient Eduardo, a grossly obese contractor, complained of daytime sleepiness to the point where he fell asleep at the wheel while driving his workers home. At the crucial moment, they screamed in fear, waking him just before he ran off the road. He was so disturbed by what happened that he swore never again to drive when he was tired. Unfortunately, he was still tired most of the time. Once we determined he had a sleep problem in part due to his massive weight, he started an antidepressant that not only helped him stay awake but also reduced his appetite. Ultimately Ed was able to lose over a hundred pounds and no longer gets drowsy behind the wheel.

Sleep disorders are commonly associated with depression. People, who are depressed, wake up with abnormally low cortisol that slowly creeps up as the day advances. This is why depressed patients usually say they feel terrible in the morning but might improve as the day goes on. Unluckily, constant unremitting stress upsets the normal cortisol cycle, reversing its circadian pattern. In the long run, the highest cortisol levels are reached during the night, completely putting a stop to deep sleep and creating more fatigue. This vicious cycle of poor sleep and daytime tiredness permanently disturbs the timing of peak cortisol levels, which is crucial for normal mental functioning. This is why depressed people cannot focus or concentrate.

Current research shows the group of most concern these days is obese adolescents or adults with obstructive sleep apnea (snoring and sleep-related breathing difficulties). A shortage of oxygen or excess of carbon dioxide can aggravate this condition, which can become life threatening. Both estrogen and progesterone seem to protect women from this severe type of sleep-disordered breathing.

What's more, progesterone therapy has brought positive results to men who snore, much to the relief of their sleep partners. Progesterone is a neurosteroid and plays a curious role in regulating body temperature. Cold hands and cold feet may thus be due, in part, to a progesterone deficiency. Another added benefit is that true progesterone helps protect arteries from thickening as a result of Type II diabetes and may help regulate cholesterol levels.

Like most hormones, progesterone levels drop with age. Some of the negative results of this actual decline could be overcome with appropriate use of progesterone supplements. Considering all of the beneficial factors, I believe that therapy with progesterone, the mother of all hormones, can prove an effective tool either as a vaginal gel, transdermal cream or capsule, to help maintain and restore hormonal balance.

What Are Phytoestrogens and How Do They Work?

Phytoestrogens are plant-based compounds that can supposedly bind to the estrogen receptor, blocking excess estrogen activity. They have a similar configuration to the estradiol molecule but their estrogenic activity is a thousand times less. Rarely, these compounds can halt the occurrence of hot flashes, decrease bone loss and reduce the risk of breast cancer in a few women. In clinical studies, surprisingly, most of the results were no better than placebo, but all the research is not yet in.

Phytoestrogens are extracted from soybeans and sold as "isoflavones," over-the -counter and these seem safer and more *unadulterated* than some pharmaceutical agents. For example, Japanese women, who generally experience one-sixth the incidence of breast cancer as compared to Western women, eat larger quantities of soy in their diet.

Soy is considered a crude blocker of environmental estrogens and contains both genistein and daidzein flavinoids. Red clover is another rich source of bioactive isoflavones and was found to be superior to placebo in reducing the symptoms of hot flushes and night sweats. Promensil®, by Novagen, in a dose of 80 milligrams resulted in a significant reduction in hot flushes by 44 percent.

Black cohosh, also known by either its scientific names (Actaea racemosa and Cimicifuga racemosa) is a member of the buttercup family native to the Eastern United States. The roots and rhizomes of the herb have a long history of use by Native American tribes to deal with urinary complaints in women. An extract of black cohosh has been used in German clinical practice since the mid-1950s with safe and effective results. Cohosh has been approved by the German government as nonprescription medication for the treatment of menopausal symptoms as Remifemin® manufactured by Enzymatic Therapy.

Black cohosh has become increasingly popular as the most widely used organic alternative to hormone replacement therapy (HRT). The herb's popularity with middle-aged women and gynecologists grew significantly after the summer of 2003 when the WHI government-sponsored clinical study on HRT was halted prematurely.

Some women normally have low levels of hormones in their bodies. Asian women, for example, have much lower levels of female hormones than African American women and also develop osteoporosis more frequently. Asian women have a lower incidence of breast and uterine cancers. The reasons for a woman's individual response to hormone therapy are varied. Differences may be due to variation in the absorption of estrogen and progestins or the distribution of estrogen receptors in the patient's estrogen-responsive organs. Again, I want to stress that both diet and the intake of phytoestrogens may play a role in the activity of estrogen receptors, but this has not yet been proven.

Why Are There So Many Different Hormone Preparations?

Women often ask me, "Why are there so many different estrogen preparations?" The clinical message is clear: each woman responds uniquely to a given dose and delivery of estrogen therapy. For this reason, treatment should be tailored to the individual woman, as it is for men. Response will vary greatly depending on the organ systems involved and the existing balance of hormones.

Technology now provides a distinction between "healthy women" who are experiencing a reproductive transition and "patients" who have hidden disease. This biologic evidence-based approach allows doctors of medicine to decide on the need for hormone therapy, the dose that should be prescribed and the patient's response to her treatment over time. A number of therapeutic options are available. Treating all women with the same dose of replacement therapy deprives women of the right to personalized care.

In the shift from synthetic estrogens, new non-synthetic testosterone patches and pure estrogen gels for women are in the works and some will soon receive FDA approval. BioSante's estrogen gel, Bio-E®, is in the final stages of FDA approval as of the writing of this book and Solvay's estrogen, EstroGel®, has already been approved for market. The future looks bright for a safer, more effective hormone treatment incorporating bioidentical hormones in a form that can be safely applied directly to the skin for both men and women.

Now that we have reviewed estrogen treatments for women, we need to look at another group of compounds that could stimulate your male partner's appreciation of bioidentical hormones.

Toxic and Intoxicating—What's the Difference?

The difference between "toxic" and "intoxicating" is that a "toxic" substance is harmful, while an "intoxicating" one is addictive. Pesticides are an example of toxic items. They are deadly to the pests we want to destroy, but we probably won't get hooked on swallowing pesticides. They are toxic, but not intoxicating.

Intoxicating substances create insatiable desires for more of the substance and can damage hormones. The most common intoxicants in our culture are illegal drugs like cocaine and speed and some legal drugs such as alcohol and caffeine. Any mind-altering medicine or herb, including prescription drugs, can become intoxicating if it creates feelings of pleasure.

The intoxicating effects of drugs are harmful to pregnant women and children, but doubly injurious to the developing embryo because it is at the most delicate life stage. When the cells in mother's womb are reproducing and joining together, the developing life form is extremely sensitive to drugs, alcohol and other harmful substances.

The emerging endocrine system distributes hormones throughout the fetus, playing a vital role in the baby's normal development. At this vulnerable stage of life, tiny amounts of toxic compounds can easily disrupt hormones. Possible consequences include: improperly formed genital organs, infertility, cancer and dozens of other health problems. It may be years before you suffer the consequences of pre-birth exposure to these substances, but they will eventually leave their mark.

We need to consider the embryo when we talk to the public about the growth and development of the child. Theo Colborn, noted author and expert on how hormones are disrupted, points out that the federal government's new Children's Health Initiative talks about the child from the day it is born through puberty but doesn't mention prenatal exposure to toxins, apparently because of possible association with the abortion issue.

This is unfortunate, because of the embryo's exquisite susceptibility to exposure to toxins. The unborn baby is incapable of defending itself against these substances, spelling tragedy for the growing child. "During embryonic and fetal development, the brain isn't developed thus far, so you've got an individual that has no feedback mechanism to protect it. The fetus is still growing new tissue, constructing its nervous system, constructing elements of its immune system and the reproductive tract." As an adult, Colborn says, "when all your organs are formed and fully functioning, it takes a lot more to blow them away," and blow them away we do on a daily basis.

Most chemicals that are toxic to insects are weakly estrogenic. This means they mimic the action of estrogen in the human body to some extent. Too much of this effect upsets the normal ratio between testosterone and estrogen in the system. Common products such as insect spray, weed killer, PVC pipe, plastic wrap, furniture finishes and baby bottles contain low amounts of toxic chemicals. For years we assumed that the toxicity of these items was so low that it had little effect on human health.

Now we're having second thoughts. By studying all of these substances collectively, we find that the way these chemical mixtures interact with the estrogen receptor and the androgen receptor have profound biological implications.

A number of chemicals used in animal food products have estrogenic activity. Since these chemicals rapidly cross the placenta, exposure to these chemicals adds to the total amount of estrogen to which a fetus is exposed. At extremely low maternal doses, these chemicals disrupt the developing endocrine system.

In the US we release more than 60 million pounds of chemicals into our water, air and soil every year. This works out to about 28 pounds of chemicals for each person in the United States on an annual basis. These chemicals can disturb our physiology, including our endocrine systems and lead to cancer, increased organ failures, poorly functioning ovaries, reduced sperm count and lower fertility rates. Babies born after exposure in the womb, have a higher probability of birth defects, certain diseases, such as diabetes, asthma, arthritis, heart disease and a lower birth weight.

The hazards of insecticides were first made known to the public in Rachel Carson's *Silent Spring,* written in 1962. A writer for the US Fish and Wildlife Service, Carson was disturbed by the nation's widespread use of chemical pesticides. After resigning from her government career in 1952, she became the world's first environmentalist. Carson theorized that human beings are a vulnerable part of the ecosystem and are threatened by the increasing use of harmful substances in the environment. Her work influenced environmental policy, leading eventually to the total US ban of DDT in 1972. Until that time, DDT, or dichlorodiphenyltrichloroethane, was the most widely used insecticide in the country.

Unfortunately, chemicals like DDT take many years, perhaps centuries, to degrade. So persistent is DDT in the environment that the bodies of penguins in Antarctica and Arctic seals and frogs living at high altitudes in remote regions are all found to contain DDT.

In 2001 a comprehensive study of heavily industrialized communities found that residents of these communities were experiencing an increase in reproductive or developmental defects. The factories in the areas produced manufactured toxins in high volume. This problem has become quite serious in countries like Japan and China where few regulations exist to limit environmental pollution.

Eight years prior to that study, a research project reported in the prestigious British medical journal, *Lancet,* examined the effects of excess estrogen on sperm. Their study suggested a cause-and-effect relationship between estrogenic chemicals and declines in human sperm counts and an increase in abnormal sperm. In addition, exposure of pregnant women to these chemicals was linked to higher rates of cancer and malformations of the penis and testicles in their male babies.

Another study by French and Argentinean researchers added further evidence to the case against environmental toxins. Argentinean men who had attended an infertility clinic between 1995 and 1998 were quizzed about their lifestyle, medical history, occupation and exposure to pesticides. The scientists concluded that being exposed to pesticides might have been a factor in the men's inability to have children. Men exposed to these chemicals were more likely to have sperm levels well below the minimum limit for male fertility or decreased motility. They also had higher levels of abnormal sperm and female sex hormones in their system than men who had not come into contact with these chemicals.

At high doses, these endocrine disruptive chemicals or EDCs cause an increase in prostate size. Dioxin is persistent and ubiquitous (present everywhere) while it accumulates in fat cells. It has the potential for decreasing masculinity and increasing feminine sexual behavior in men. Exposure to dioxin at birth leads to long-lasting effects over a wide range of brain functions including posttraumatic stress disorder and attention deficit disorder.

Our growing dependence on intoxicating drugs adds to the load of toxic waste in our bodies and brains. Over 36 million Americans regularly use the two most powerful legal drugs known to mankind: nicotine and alcohol. Habitual use of these and other legal drugs contributes dramatically to sexual dysfunction in America. A dangerous stew results when drugs and pesticides commingle in the human body. This combination disrupts the sensitive hormonal balance of entire populations.

The Anti-aphrodisiacs—Alcohol and Nicotine

Tobacco and alcohol abuse have a negative effect on sperm levels, libido and overall health. Cigarettes often act as a "gateway drug" leading to the abuse of other drugs. The longer anyone uses alcohol, marijuana or nicotine, the lower his or her level of testosterone drops and the higher estrogen rises. I am certain you have not seen this on any warning labels on cigarettes or alcohol, but this might explain the sex-destroying effect of these what I call "*anti-aphrodisiacs.*"

Nicotine accelerates tolerance, physical dependence and withdrawal symptoms more quickly than any other drug known to man. Nicotine exposure in young men can lead to shrinking of the testicles, impaired sperm formation, poor semen quality and a lower count of total and living sperm.

Nevertheless many people resist giving up drug habits that are so harmful to their hormones, minds and bodies because addiction is stronger than common sense. Health is neglected in the minds of those who are unhappy, stressed out or depressed, relying on drugs to get them through the day. Addiction affects over ten percent of the American population and its victims fill our hospital wards.

Furthermore the consequences of legal drug abuse include a weakened immune system and a heightened risk of heart disease, stroke and cancer in both sexes. Prolonged reliance on toxic drugs can result in lung or liver disease and enlarged breast tissue in men. It is a shame that many health problems associated with drug use do not become obvious until later in life when it is too late to reverse their effects.

Not long ago cigarette companies were claiming that their products were safe and that consumers were responsible for choosing to become dependent. Losing their first class action suit was a wake-up call. Their defense faded away following strong language by the Surgeon General's report in 1999 stating that, "…nicotine is the most addictive substance known to man." People who stop using nicotine experience severe withdrawal symptoms, sensations like a rat gnawing in their stomach, irritability, anxiety, and difficulty concentrating along with increased appetite and sleep disturbances. It is not easy to quit smoking, so why start?

Lung cancer and emphysema are well known health problems associated with heavy cigarette smoking. Tar and other pollutants in the smoke of cigarettes can initiate these illnesses but it takes decades (about twenty years) for the harmful effects to be noticed. The real culprit, however, is nicotine, the powerful, habit-forming drug that can create dependence after only a few exposures.

We are just beginning to realize the devastating effects of this poison in our society. The nicotine in five cigarettes is sufficient to paralyze and kill most animals. Toxins in nicotine and other pesticides including dioxin, threaten our hormonal balance and normal sexual functioning.

Most smokers never imagine the consequences of their habit on their sex life. They are lulled into a sense of complacency and a deceptive belief that "it won't happen to me." Yet studies show that smoking is the *number one* cause of erectile dysfunction in the Western world. Prolonged use of our popular drugs such as alcohol, marijuana and nicotine decrease both testosterone and DHT levels. Certain high blood pressure pills, fungicidal medications, acid suppressors and over-the-counter pain pills also lower testosterone levels.

The alarming fact that nicotine has the potential of rendering entire segments of our population impotent and sterile should be stressed. We need to wake up and stop pretending that smoking doesn't affect our sexual performance and reproductive abilities. Women must realize that they can become addicted to nicotine and alcohol more easily than men. They have a reduced tolerance and often a *single exposure* can create a *lifetime of dependence*.

It has been pointed out that cigarettes are the only product legally manufactured and advertised in the United States that, when used as directed, will cause death and disease. The rate of addiction among regular cigarette smokers aged 24 and younger is rising though the overall popularity of smoking has dropped. Younger smokers have a stronger tendency to become addicted than those who are older. In addition, the sexual maturation of the male is very sensitive to hormones and environmental toxins.

These poisons cause damaged sperm cells and reduced numbers of sperm, lower quality of sperm and less capacity of the sperm to penetrate or fertilize the egg. Sperm with DNA damage usually have a lower fertilization rate and may be the reason for the delay in impregnation routinely seen in smokers. In the early stages of life, the risk of cell damage from smoking and other environmental hazards emerges more often in males than in females. David, the patient who visited me, had been smoking since the age of twelve.

Here is more bad news! In either sex, smoking can also damage the blood-clotting factors or platelets, causing increased blood clotting when it is not desirable and possibly leading to a stroke. "Is coffee bad in the morning?" is a question I often hear. Well the use of more than 500 milligrams of caffeine, the amount in *four cups* of coffee, gives rise to neck aches, headaches, trouble sleeping and higher blood pressure in women. Drinking more than four cups of coffee and smoking more than one pack of cigarettes can kill off sperm, increase abnormal forms and decrease sperm motility. At these same rates, women develop a decrease of vaginal secretions and clitoral sensitivity.

What about cigar smoking? Many people assume that cigar smoking doesn't pose a significant health risk since cigar smoke isn't inhaled to the same degree as cigarette smoke. Alas, these cigar smokers are deluded. Lung disease may not be as common among cigar smokers, but they are likely to encounter circulatory or heart-related health problems from poisons that are absorbed through the lining of the mouth. Carlos Iribarren, at Kaiser Permanente in Oakland, California underscored the dangers of cigar smoking, in a 1998 study. The overall death rate among cigar smokers was found to be 25 percent *higher* than the rate for non-smokers. Smokers using an alcohol-based mouthwash increase their incidence of mouth and throat cancer many times over.

The perils of smoking are drawing the attention of our country's leaders as never before. For the first time our government's "top doctor," Surgeon General Richard H. Carmona said publicly, in 1999 that he supported the banning of all tobacco products. If smoking were eliminated, the health of the population would increase fourfold and most smokers' anxiety would disappear. Doctors estimate that 50% of the anxiety in our population is related to smoking the stimulant nicotine. Why don't we pay attention?

The Combination of Social Lubricants-Party Time!

When Shakespeare said, "Drink increaseth the desire and decreaseth the performance," he didn't realize how right he was. For men, a moderate amount of alcohol is considered to be about one ounce of pure alcohol per day. That is equivalent to two beers, two glasses of wine or two shots of whisky. Yes, they each contain the same amount of pure ethanol. For women, half that amount is considered a moderate consumption because women are *twice as sensitive* to alcohol as men. Only three drinks per week is the recommended limit for women to reduce the risk of breast cancer. Ideally, women at risk for breast cancer should *never* drink.

The wine industry spends a chunk of their advertising budget promoting the consumption of wine as a way to reduce the risk of heart disease. The popular press has echoed their claims, giving considerable attention to the favorable effects of alcohol on the heart. To date, there are no controlled trials to prove this beneficial effect. There is some evidence that certain antioxidants in grape juice may be protective of the heart but alcohol itself is toxic to heart muscle. As far as sexual health is concerned, it's far worse. Studies indicate that past heavy drinking is definitely associated with a reduction in testosterone.

When men combine nicotine, alcohol and anti-hypertensive medications they sometimes notice the loss of erections and premature impotence. For women, the deadly-combo increases breast cancer risk along with an entire range of diseases including cirrhosis of the liver, kidney failure, heart attacks and emphysema. For many 60-year-old men, the previous abuse of alcohol and nicotine has a much greater impact on their sexual function than aging or environmental estrogens.

Some middle-aged men are unknowingly affected by alcohol-induced hypogonadism, a condition marked by an impaired production of testosterone. It becomes easy to see that many men are creating their own problems by abusing legal drugs. Several physicians do not stress the relationship of these drug habits to their patients' hormones. It is usually left up to the wives or girlfriends to point out the connection.

Remember that any man may develop greater tolerance to alcohol or other drugs over time but he may not notice a problem with erections until his intake of alcohol becomes excessive. Binge drinking can bring out a hormonal insufficiency at an earlier age.

As mentioned, women also become easily addicted to alcohol. An early sign of dependence in women, subsequent to the loss of their sexual dreams, is the avoidance of quality female friendships. Women tend to experience a diminished ability to reason, once they become addicted to any intoxicant. Since women are likely to do the bulk of the shopping, the liquor industry focuses it's advertising on them. As a doctor I make it a point to discuss this problem with all my patients, because it's important for women to realize that they are not helping their men by buying liquor and serving it or stocking up the refrigerator.

Alcoholism is an enormous problem creating most of the deaths on the road. Then too, teenagers and new drivers, inexperienced in handling a car, already have the highest rate of traffic accidents in the country. Did you know that by one estimate, half the admissions to hospitals are alcohol related? If you doubt my word, drop by your local emergency room and see how many patients are the victims of alcohol-related accidents, fights or over-consumption. For these sufferers, impotence is the least of their problem.

Tax revenue from the sale of alcohol and cigarettes makes politicians important advocates for these two industries. Can you believe that at a time when governments banned smoking in restaurants and bars in California, most cities in middle America still don't have "no smoking" ordinances that effectively protect the rights of their citizens? Lobbyists working for international corporations defend the legality of the two most abused drugs in our society—alcohol and tobacco.

The American government has yielded to financial and political pressures to protect industries that are damaging the health of the American public. Our government leaders should stop promoting lofty goals for tomorrow's populace and start listening to the symptoms of poor health and loss of reproductive capacity among its citizens. Do you think that the US government will ever outlaw alcohol and tobacco the way they outlaw marijuana? Would that be a good idea?

The sad reality is that Americans love their drugs and that devotion will not disappear on its own. Rich and poor alike will continue to abuse their health by using excessive amounts of illegal and hazardous legal drugs for their intoxicating effects.

Drunk drivers are still the leading cause of death on the road.

Cigarettes and alcohol are traditional social lubricants; giving rise to the popularity of drinking and smoking among our youth. At parties, bars or at home and on the street, in states where smoking is still permitted in bars, a cigarette or a glass of whisky is an undemanding prop for those who are nervous about what to do with their hands.

Drinkers and smokers have an increased tendency to develop elevated blood pressure, heart disease and impotence. Testosterone is only the first victim of our nonchalance about the abuse of legalized intoxicating drugs in the United States. Let's listen to these warnings and take steps to curtail the delivery of toxic products to the mothers, fathers and future generations of our society. If you or your spouse smoke, quit at once and if you have already quit, congratulate yourself on the improvement in health you will continue to experience.

As a means of pressuring men to avoid the adverse consequences of alcohol abuse, I often urge them to stop drinking for a specific time period. This is the most effective type of preventive medical intervention. In addition to that, there is a simple and effective way to eliminate the effect of the toxic contaminants—avoid smoking and drinking completely. This is not easy in a society where the use of these products is not only legal but actively promoted. The advertising budget of the tobacco industry alone exceeds the gross national income of many countries.

Our government considers the economic losses, measured by lost jobs and revenues, as too great to risk if they were to limit the industries that deliver these poisonous substances to our citizenry. You may wonder why these substances are so toxic. What's in a cigarette that's so bad? Is it just the nicotine or the smoke?

Dioxin, the Most Toxic Substance Known to Man

What is dioxin? Dioxin is the most deadly substance on the earth. The manufacturing of vinyl is the leading source of dioxin in the US environment. That's correct, the most toxic substance in the world is used to make credit cards and vinyl blinds. Vinyl is a plastic material used in house siding, windows, PVC pipes, medical packaging and credit cards. Vinyl makes it possible to own beautiful and inexpensive dishes and glasses. Many kitchen appliances, windows, furniture and even some food containers are coated with vinyl.

Unluckily, when vinyl breaks down, as it inevitably does over time or when it is heated or burned, it releases dioxin *directly* into the environment. When you cover food with a plastic wrap and turn on the microwave, dioxin can literally drip onto your food from the sheets of protective plastic. Your old computers and scanners contribute a deadly stream of dioxin into the aquifer as they break down over time in our landfills.

Tip: Recycle all your old cell phones, phones, computers, engine oils and plastics.

Dioxins are the unintended by-product of any process involving the burning of compound with high chlorine content. Dioxin is present in the smoke that comes from either end of a cigarette. That means that *second hand smoke* and smoke from the filtered end of a cigarette is loaded with dioxin. The chemical name of the most common dioxin is tetrachlorodibenzodioxin or TCDD for short.

Nobody manufactures dioxins on purpose. The major contributors of dioxin are pesticides, wood preservatives and the burning of fossil fuels such as gasoline and waste incinerator or engine oil. As mentioned, the more heavily industrialized countries have the worst problems with dioxin. Furthermore, countries where smoking is allowed on the streets have much higher dioxin levels in their air. This situation contributes to asthma and respiratory diseases.

Globally, dioxin pollutants endure without restriction in many countries. The dioxin-producing pesticide DDT is still used in South America and Africa. Regrettably, dioxin is also a major factor contributing to infertility in men who spray DDT to control the spread of malaria in Africa.

Dioxin oozes from the siding of houses and is mixed into furniture and appliances. Subsequently, it filters into water and soil, contaminating the food chain. The dioxin you absorb from foods enters your body when you eat contaminated fats and meat by-products. Fortunately, your liver is able to detoxify much of this poison by tucking it away in your body's fat stores. Dioxin has a major effect on your testosterone availability by disrupting hormone levels and leading to a serious deficiency.

This powerful hormone-disrupting chemical has become associated with an epidemic of testosterone deficiency. Testosterone deficiencies interfere with normal sexual development in males and females, affecting fertility. The problem of infertility has spread to most of the Western and industrialized world. Future generations may be affected with a lower birthrate after being exposed to dioxin as children before or after birth.

A fertility rate of 2.1 births per woman is needed to maintain population levels. Instead, the U.S. rate hovers around 2.0 births per woman and in Europe has dropped to 1.42. Yet in less developed countries where the impact on the population of a high birthrate is modified by high infant mortality rates and a short lifespan, the birthrate has dropped from 6.2 to 3.0 births per woman over the past 30 years.

As a result of these trends, over the past four years the United Nations has reduced its projections for the world's total population in 2050 from 9.8 billion people to 8.9 billion. Almost a billion less people than we thought. Experts estimate that another billion will be cut from the estimates within a few years. Does this represent a desirable form of population control?

Environmental estrogen pollution has become a worldwide problem producing low sperm counts, miscarriages and reproductive disorders. Babies exposed to dioxins before birth are more likely to have a lower IQ, learning disabilities, a short attention span and damaged immune and nervous systems. Contamination from dioxin leads to a higher risk of attention deficit disorder (ADD), asthma, allergies, diabetes, endometriosis and miscarriages. These problems have reached critical mass for all peoples living on our planet.

The failure of world leaders to take this threat seriously endangers the survival of our planet's population. The delicately balanced hormonal system that has evolved, unchanged over eons, is in danger of being damaged beyond hope of repair.

How Can We Stop Poisoning Ourselves?

Dioxin is still the most deadly substance on the planet. Making its debut in the American consciousness as the herbicide "Agent Orange", dioxin was used as a defoliant in the Vietnam war. The EPA is overwhelmed by the enormity of trying to control dioxin because it is toxic at a dilution of less than five parts per trillion. This pollutant persists for decades. We must all pay attention to our environment and do something about it while we still have a chance.

How can Americans protect themselves against pesticide and dioxin exposure? One way would be to stay indoors and stop buying poisons to store under your sink. Or you can wear gas masks during dust storm activity when chemicals waft your way along the jet stream from Asia, or you could eat only plants and avoid all animal fats where most of the dioxin is concentrated. You could stop smoking, drinking or using pesticides. None of these would help much since toxins have permeated every aspect of your lifestyle! Let me give you an example of how dioxin might affect a typical American couple.

Peter, a 36 year-old salesman, could not grasp why Jean, his wife of many years was complaining so much. Jean, only 38 years old, wondered why her husband had stopped being the aggressive, fun-loving sex partner she'd married 11 years earlier. It seemed he hardly ever started things rolling toward a sexually enlivening experience. If she insisted, he went along—and achieved an erection—but he didn't seem to care whether she had an orgasm or not, immediately turning his back to her after sex. Peter used to be a great lover. What happened?

Puzzled, Jean wondered if Pete, an agricultural specialist, was getting too much exposure from bug sprays and other pesticides in his work. He was too macho to wear protective clothing or any breathing apparatus. She was becoming concerned. She decided to try to convince her husband to see a doctor. If he agreed and if the doctor ordered the tests that confirmed a toxic exposure or excess estrogens, something could still be done. What is it about these toxins from pesticides that affected Peter? Could they lower your partner's libido too?

Endocrine Disruptive Chemicals

Mankind's poisons include toxins, pesticides, herbicides, fungicides and heavy metals. These endocrine disruptive chemicals or EDCs have the ability to stimulate the estrogen receptors. In particular, too much dioxin can haphazardly alter the entire testosterone pathway in your body. Dioxin literally blocks the formation of many hormones creating an irreversible hormone insufficiency. Each one of these disruptions is related to the estrogen-like activity of these substances. EDCs disturb both human and animal endocrine systems.

Straying into the human system from polluted air and water, these foreign estrogens have been found in concentrations measured in parts per million to parts per billion. At such microscopic levels, they were once considered safe. Now we know that environmental estrogens are toxic at extremely low concentrations, measured in parts per *trillion*. This means that the risk of harmful symptoms from EDCs is thousands to millions of times greater than we used to think.

A new batch of pollutants, a different group of hormone-like chemicals, is currently threatening your husbands' or boyfriends' testosterone levels. These newly discovered organic molecules dubbed *phthalates* are a relative of the dioxin molecule but are far removed from insecticides or fungicides. Most Americans use them on a daily basis.

Phthalates are everywhere in our surroundings. Phthalates are routinely used in personal care products such as soaps and shampoos and in medical products like tubing or plastics to keep them soft and flexible. Tests for phthalates on human urine samples from across our country demonstrate levels that exceed safe or acceptable levels. The levels were highest in women for two phthalate solvents used in American cosmetics, hair dyes, fingernail polish, paints and soft plastic containers. In this instance, women are at higher risk. Undoubtedly, all plastic dishes, containers and plastic grocery bags contain phthalates.

How do phthalates affect testosterone levels? You may recall that when testosterone converts to DHT or dihydrotestosterone at puberty, it exerts masculinizing effects on boys and triggers estrogen release in girls. DHT initiates the onset of puberty: stimulating penis development, sexual drive and other bodily changes. Obviously DHT is quite an important hormone.

As boys become adolescents, dihydrotestosterone (DHT) increases muscular strength and brings about the deepening of the voice, the growth of facial hair and enlargement of sexual organs. DHT increases a girl's interest in boys as they enter puberty, making it an essential part of the life cycle. Phthalates totally block this androgen receptor effect in both sexes. Prenatal exposure to phthalates and other EDCs also affects genital development in babies.

Studies indicate that phthalates can interfere with sex hormones and impair reproductive health by directly blocking the action of DHT on the androgen receptor. Researchers at the Harvard School of Public Health in Boston found phthalates in both semen and urine samples of at least 75 percent of volunteers attending a clinic for couples experiencing difficulty conceiving a child. Could there be a connection?

Phthalate and dioxin exposures have devastating effects on both young men and young women. By acting as a potent estrogen, EDCs feminize males, creating problems in sexual function and in the ultimate size of their sexual organs. To offset these negative effects, early testosterone monitoring and supplementation is necessary if we are to restore fertility and normal sexual function in those affected.

Mature sperm counts climb in order to make reproduction possible. Phthalates interfere with this process by both decreasing sperm counts and sperm maturation. Authors of a study from the journal *Epidemiology* in May of 2003 believe that dioxin exposure and the presence of phthalates could explain why semen quality is *declining worldwide*. But there are other EDCs that have more profound hormonal effects.

Furthermore, environmental estrogens and androgens may be the major contributors to the *pandemic* of breast, uterine and prostate cancers around the world. Estrogen-like compounds are not the only problem. Excess male hormones can duplicate the action of testosterone as they seep into the rivers and streams in runoff from pulp and paper mills. These testosterone-like compounds affect fish and frogs by masculinizing the females. Fake hormones are all around us! Fake androgens can even create precocious or premature puberty in young boys.

An excess of DHT in the water around these old paper mills has been implicated in other changes. Sex ratios in fish change dramatically with more males born than females giving rise to endangered species. Herbicides in rainwater, usually estrogen-like, feminize male frogs. It's not only mercury contamination in fish that is dangerous. Fish in the Great Lakes have been found with both testicles and ovarian tissue. Excess androgens may be masculinizing females in our society while estrogens are feminizing males. This is an insupportable arrangement for *equalization of the sexes*.

It gets worse as active forms of several hormones are being detected in sewage wastes dumped into the oceans, eaten by fish and subsequently consumed by the public. When such affected fish are used as feed at "salmon farms," they increase the levels of pollutants in the tissues of farmed fish. Farmed salmon in Norway have been found to contain *three times* the amount of dioxin and *thirty times* the amount of PCBs of wild salmon. Because they are fed artificially with contaminated fish, EDCs are concentrated in their fat cells. If you eat these fish, the same thing happens.

While you cannot totally avoid these toxins, you can minimize their potential effect by eliminating foods containing animal fats, including farmed fish. Of course, vegetarianism is always an option. In the majority of cases this means increasing complex carbohydrates, which is easily achieved by following a plant-based diet. But the idea of becoming a vegetarian does not appeal to everybody.

Many Americans are looking to low carbohydrate and high animal protein diets to help them lose weight. These types of diets have been found to be the *least nutritious* of any diet plan and lead to the greatest disruption in metabolism. They can lead to diabetes, osteoporosis and heart disease.

Andrew Weil, author of *Eating Well for Optimum Health: The Essential guide to Food, Diet, and Nutrition,* said it very well. "The nation is in the grip of low-carb mania, the latest dietary craze. It is important for people to understand than an optimum diet includes a balance of carbohydrates, fats and protein. Carbohydrates are not bad foods anymore than fats are. It is important for people to understand, however, that there are good and bad carbohydrate foods, good and bad fats and better and worse protein choices."

Chef-prepared meats and fish are considered a tasty treat among our citizens. Fresh fish tastes great, especially raw. But watch out for mercury contamination! Avoid uncooked fish in sushi bars; tuna may taste great but these fish contain mercury and dioxins. Cooking destroys 50 percent of the dioxin in food, but foods cooked in the microwave in plastic containers or covered with plastic wrap can release toxins directly into your foods. Microwaves are safe; it's the containers that are dangerous.

At this time, there is no such thing as a "safe" microwaveable plastic wrap, although the plastic industry is now promoting this feature.

The best solution is to use only ceramic or glass dishes in the microwave oven. For similar reasons, plastic dishes and glasses should not be used for hot foods or foods with a high acid content. Acid and heat can leach toxins directly from the plastic itself. In some cases simply storing food in some plastics is enough to absorb dioxin.

So what is the solution? In spite of eating a totally plant-based diet, it would still be impossible to avoid the plentiful plastics and cosmetics in our world. But eating foods lower in the food chain definitely reduces your total exposure to these lethal chemicals. It takes real commitment to modify your diet and your lifestyle but the results are worth it.

Once again I offer sound advice from Dr. Weil, "We recommend that people decrease consumption of the following foods: foods of animal origin (other than fish), refined and processed foods, fast food, high-glycemic-load carbohydrates, and polyunsaturated vegetable oils. We recommend that they eliminate margarine, vegetable shortening, and products made with partially hydrogenated oils."

Women, who usually control food shopping, can take a big step in protecting themselves from harmful chemicals by decreasing their exposure especially during pregnancy. Healthy and safe cosmetic products including: lipstick, face cream and makeup removers are available if you make the effort to find them. The use of cosmetics such as hair dyes and fingernail polish is a choice, not a necessity. We can each choose healthy alternatives to cosmetics, processed foods or to farmed animals.

There are other things you can do, too. Dr. Weil encourages organic food choices. "We strongly support organic agriculture and better production, distribution and marketing of organic produce to make it available and affordable to more people." Organic foods, including meats from animals raised organically, are now widely available in American supermarkets. Another way to enjoy good food that is free from harmful poisons is to select fresh fruits and vegetables grown organically.

Antioxidants and other plant-based phytochemicals are also helpful in stopping the harmful effects of EDCs in the diet. When used in conjunction with the beneficial bioflavinoids in fresh fruits, seeds, nuts and vegetables, anti-oxidant vitamins can remove bioactive compounds, which initiate DNA mutations and tissue damage. Vitamins A, C and E are a few of the antioxidant vitamins, but locally grown fruits and vegetables are still the best reservoir of these beneficial antioxidants and phytonutrients.

The health of your children is worth the small extra cost of organic products or supplemental hormone therapy. Your future fertility and the lives of your descendants are in your hands. You need to do more to let your government representatives know that to protect your children and your fertility, all Americans must have air, water and meat that are free from contaminants.

Meat, Crucial for the Development of Man

"Let thy food be thy medicine and thy medicine be thy food."
—Hippocrates (460-377 BC)

Our need to survive influenced our biology. Primitive peoples hunted animals to supplement the diet of nuts and berries that they could forage. Women, who excelled in verbal ability, probably developed language to communicate with their children. Or, perhaps spoken communication was developed among men, in order to improve their hunting strategies. Still, gender differences were based on the hunter-gatherer lifestyle, with men trained for the hunt and women for cooking and serving food. At the dawn of mankind, high-quality protein, in the form of hunted meat, made a definite contribution to the growth and refinement of the brain.

On the plains and grasslands of the African savannah, primitive man developed the skills needed to hunt animals. Mankind would not have evolved to this point were it not for the cooperation of these early humans in their quest for meat. Meat continues to play an important role in the diets of many people in "Westernized" countries and for those who can afford it, meat is often the primary source of food.

In the early days of hunting and gathering for food, meat was a quick and easy supply of nutritious protein. The high protein load from killed animals apparently helped man's brain to grow and hunting probably helped early humans to advance socially and physically.

Man continues to evolve today, still using animals for food, but the continued development of the brain no longer requires the proteins of animal fleshy tissue. The reality is that we do not have to eat meat any longer. A growing number of people around the world feel for religious and other reasons that the flesh of animals should not be consumed as food; for millions of others on the planet, eating meat is just not an economical choice.

Today livestock are kept in horrendous conditions and are often sick and infected. Antibiotics are used routinely, often mixed into every meal the animals eat, simply to keep them alive in their crowded feedlots or cages. As a result of this practice, bacteria that are resistant to antibiotics have evolved, threatening the health of the animals and humans.

There are other parts of animals raised for food that affect our health. You should never eat the brains of any animal. You should avoid all organ meats because these are the body parts most likely to be contaminated with environmental toxins. There are certain brain proteins identified as "prions," which can reproduce themselves in people and initiate *mad cow disease* or other degenerative nervous conditions.

The first case of "mad cow disease" in the US was discovered at the end of 2003 in an infected cow in Washington State. The government quickly determined that it came from Canada and blocked all meat imports. The second case was identified in a US feedlot late in 2004 and reported to the public in June of 2005. The third case was reported in July of 2005. Apparently these two cows were kept out of the food chain but it seems suspicious that it took six months and three confirmatory tests to identify the problem. During this time, infected cows mingled freely and may have spread the disease. In Britain and France, when mad cow was detected, millions of cattle were destroyed. To this day, most European countries *will not* import American beef.

Ironically, those cows in the US that were fed body parts of other animals are strict vegetarians that would eat only grass if allowed to graze at will. The adulteration of beef from the feeding of entrails to cows created the environment for mad cow disease. In the wake of the mad cow scare, beef consumption has plummeted in Europe to half its former level. Yet Americans go on burying their heads in the sand like the ostrich trying to hide from its enemies. Only three infected cows have been destroyed in the US.

Killing animals for food is morally wrong for Jews, Buddhists and Hindus. But you may argue, meat is still a major part of the diet for one out of three people in the world and has been a staple in the human diet for centuries. A vegetarian diet is the staple pattern of eating for the remaining *two thirds* of the world population.

The ongoing waste of food involved in producing meat is another reason why meat does not make sense in today's world. About 16 pounds of grain are required to grow one pound of beef. As little as one pound of grain can make a loaf of bread. Meat is a much less efficient food than a loaf of bread. Cornell researchers have calculated that meat from the most efficient factory farm returns 34.5 percent of the fossil energy it takes to provide the meat as food energy. The *least efficient* plant food, by contrast, delivers *328 percent* as much energy as it consumes from fossil energy sources.

Another reason for avoiding meat is the tremendous amount of manure produced by animals harvested for food. A cow delivers 120 pounds of wet manure to the environment every day. Grazing livestock release 250 to 500 liters of methane gas per animal per day. Methane has 60 times as much power as carbon dioxide in contributing to the "greenhouse effect." Fortunately, methane has less impact on our weather because it only remains in the atmosphere for 10 years compared to 100 years for carbon dioxide.

Some say that meat once played a major role in the evolutionary development of intelligence, but if that is true, it does not follow that meat is essential in our diet today. Perhaps our intelligence has evolved past the point of needing to rely on meat. At the very least we should consider the fact that meat and other estrogen-laced foods, stuffed with animal fat, can be hazardous to our health, our hearts and our hormones.

But wait! Now Avian Bird Flu threatens our citizenry. This pandemic strain of influenza virus killed over 50 million people in 1918. The deadly disease is spread by wild birds and infects chickens. Millions of poultry hens have been "culled" in Asia where the pandemic started. The disease jumped from birds, to pigs and now to humans.

Not all chicken is infected with avian viruses or laced with hormone additives. It is possible to find range-fed, cage-free animal protein, organically raised without hormones and considered safer to eat. In the Jewish tradition, meat is rendered kosher—safe to eat—by killing the animal in a quick, merciful fashion and then draining all its blood. This theoretically removes all the traces of hormones released at death and the disease-causing bacteria and viruses from the meat. Salting the meat repeatedly also helps to draw out the last traces of blood, the medium in which organisms easily multiply to transmit disease. You may not be excited about asking for kosher meat, but you'll have to admit that it cuts down on the risk of blood-borne disease and the bird flu.

The *bacterial count* of meat increases exponentially from the moment of death of the animal whether it is cooked, refrigerated or frozen. By the time you consume animal protein as a hamburger, steak or chicken breast, the dead flesh has become loaded with harmful bacteria and parasites, among them salmonella, *E. coli*, trichinosis and a variety of tapeworms. John Robbins, author of, *The Food*

Revolution, asserts that in the Americas meat has become the primary cause of food-related deaths and illnesses, including heart disease caused by abnormal cholesterol readings.

In the US we keep eating meat at a level that is almost beyond belief. Meat comprises over *50 percent* of the American diet and advertising by fast food restaurants encourages higher consumption. The idea that there might be a market for a vegetarian burger is making slow progress in the restaurant business. When Burger King became the first fast food restaurant to offer a plant-based burger on its menu in 2002, the event was world news. The item did not last long.

In spite of a growing number of vegetarians in our midst—at least 12 million in the US at latest count—meat was purchased for food at the highest quantity ever in 2003. According to the US Department of Agriculture, Americans ate an average of 219 pounds of red meat, pork and poultry that year, a staggering increase of 32 percent since 1960 when the *average US citizen consumed 166 pounds* of red meat, including 64.5 pounds of beef per year.

Beef consumption in the US rose steadily in the sixties, seventies and early eighties, rising to an all time high in 1987 of 82.4 pounds per person. As a result of the tremendous amount of publicity and discussion following the 1987 publication of *Diet for a New America,* also by John Robbins, it dropped by 20 percent in the following five years and then began creeping up again.

In North America we grow enough grain products to feed the entire world. The fact that almost one half of all the corn and one third of all the grain grown we grow is used to feed and fatten animals is catastrophic. An estimated 130,000 cows and calves are slaughtered each day, according to the US Department of Agriculture. Not counting fish and other aquatic creatures, ten billion birds, animals and other creatures are slaughtered for food every year in the U.S. Fish supplies are dwindling rapidly and many birds have become extinct. What animal will appear next on the endangered species list?

Some experts like Peter Burwash, who founded an environmental group known, as "EarthSave" believe that our dependence on flesh-based diets creates most of the pollution on our planet. "Moving away from an animal based diet to a plant-based diet will decrease world pollution and decrease all chronic diseases," said EarthSave's scientific director, Dr. Michael Klapper in 1996.

We have abundant scientific evidence that animal protein is not essential for normal physiologic functioning nor is it beneficial as a source of nutrition. Since meat becomes readily polluted with environmental estrogens, it is not a leap to assume that contaminated meat is harmful to humans.

Vegetarianism—One Way to Cut Your Toxic Load

Every day we lose large chunks of earth trampled and loosened by over-grazing cattle, sheep and pigs and blown or washed out to the sea. This amounts to a net loss of about *1000 acres of topsoil per year*. Iowa has lost half its fertile topsoil over the past century and much of America is continuing to lose topsoil at an alarming rate.

When our geological resource base deteriorates as a result of topsoil depletion and pollution of our groundwater, we pass on a weakened capacity for future generations to prosper and enjoy good health. Lester Brown, president of the Earth Policy Institute, in his book *Eco-Economy* states that, "Mismanagement is destroying forests, range lands, fisheries and croplands, the four ecosystems that supply our food and, except for the minerals, all our raw materials as well. Even though many of us live in a high-tech urbanized society, we are as dependent on the earth's ecological systems as our hunter-gatherer forebears were."

Consider the decline of ancient civilizations in Mesopotamia, the Mediterranean region, Pre-Colombian southwest U.S. and Central America. Historians believe that these cultures vanished into vapor as a result of their failure to make a successful transition from subsistence farming to an agricultural economy robust enough to support large populations. Are we headed in that direction?

To help to preserve our farmland, we could alter our diet and become healthier by eating a more plant-based organic diet. Vegetarianism involves a highly rewarding lifestyle that fosters respect for oneself and other animals. In addition, most of us would lose weight on this type of diet.

Avoiding the flesh of dead animals grants us a longer lifespan, decreases chronic disease and improves our ability to control our weight. Vegetarian or not, we would all be better off if we stopped eating so many animal products. We should avoid animal fats because of the very real possibility that they are laden with deadly bugs and they contain too much dioxin.

Toxic chemicals such as dioxin affect our farm-raised animals in addition to our wildlife. Fortunately, toxic residues are not readily incorporated into many fruits, vegetables, cereal grains or other plant material, even if they are present in the soil or sprayed on the growing plant. Many pesticide residues can be washed off or peeled as the outer leaves of plants or the skin of fruit. But toxic substances are embedded in the fat of the meat tissue and cannot be removed.

Of course we can't avoid all exposure to environmental pollutants in the food chain and in our water and air, but by *modifying our food choices* we can reduce the toxic load on our bodies by almost 50 percent! As a result, we can all become happier, healthier and live longer!

Recommendations for Healthy Living

Dr. Melvyn Werbach, professor of Integrative Nutrition at Capital University wrote, "I wish to argue here that nutrition is so important to the historical development and future course of most illnesses that the patient's nutritional status should always be on the clinician's mind. Nothing is more basic to life than food and drink. Sometimes nutrition plays a predominant role in the evolution of the illness. Other times, it is not a primary etiological (causative) factor, yet nutritional therapy may still improve the clinical course." A good diet does not rule out specific nutritional deficiencies. For example, selenium is often lacking in the diet of many people and low selenium may contribute to cancer, heart disease and low fertility. Even with a good diet, dietary selenium will be low if the soil in which foods are grown is deficient.

I am going to share with you seven simple recommendations that will make it easier for you to decrease your exposure to EDCs. We would all be in better health by substituting soy for meat, consuming eggs only from free-range chickens (if at all), insisting on low-fat dairy products from organically fed cows and focusing on tofu, seeds and nuts for protein. Here are my seven recommendations for healthy living:

1. Avoid all animal fats.

Most types of animal protein, but especially organ meats, eggs, milk, cheese and margarine are high in saturated animal fats. Most of these foods are also contaminated with environmental estrogens or endocrine disruptive chemicals. If you must eat white meat, buy organic chicken without the skin and avoid farmed fish. Remove the skin and cook all fresh fish thoroughly (baking, poaching and broiling is best).

Better yet, limit your animal protein intake to dairy products with low or no fat. Dairy products can be healthy without the fat. Try to eat soybean products such as tofu, vegeburgers and tempeh instead of any meat. Books on alternative diets will give you more information on this subject. *The Accidental Vegan* by Devra Gartenstein, is a great guide to tasty meat-free vegan cooking.

2. Eat more fresh fruits, vegetables and seed oils.

Andrew Weil, a nutritional medicine expert, recommends that "people increase consumption of the following foods: fruits and vegetables, vegetable protein sources, low-glycemic-load carbohydrates (e.g., beans, whole grains, sweet potatoes, winter squashes), monounsaturated vegetable oils, nuts and seeds, and omega-3 fatty acid sources (e.g., oily fish or fish oils, walnuts, flax seeds, hemp seeds)."

These colorful foods are your best source for antioxidant vitamins and other nutrients essential for good health. Fruits and vegetables do not contain hydrogenated fat or processed sugar. Choosing healthy fats such as flaxseed, safflower, and sunflower seed, peanut, walnut, avocado, pumpkin seed, sesame and grapeseed oils, makes your meals taste better. Most seeds and nuts are also healthy options for high quality proteins and make delicious additions to salads, snacks and baked goods. Lentils, soybeans or fat-free refried beans are great protein sources and create delicious meals.

3. Stay away from saturated fats and any trans fats.
All animal tissues contain saturated fats. If you want to decrease your cholesterol levels try avoiding all fried foods, refined or artificial sugars and corn syrup as they contain various chemicals associated with an increased risk of obesity, cancer and diabetes. Commercial products such as trans fatty-acid-free Smart Balance® buttery spread or mayonnaise, sold in supermarkets and health food stores across the country, are great sources of healthy unsaturated fats. All together organic foods are delicious, convenient and better.

To avoid contamination from mercury, avoid or cut back on eating fish from the Great Lakes or any farmed salmon. Nordic Naturals (Watsonville, California) is one company that removes all the mercury plus the "fishy" taste from their fish oil capsules. When tested, most fish oils on the market were free of mercury and dioxins. For those deep-fried snacks that you hate to give up, make sure they are baked with Olestra®, an indigestible fat substitute, which could help to eliminate dioxin up to tenfold.

4. Elevate your mood by eating more foods that encourage production of serotonin and dopamine in your brain.
Bananas, tomatoes, plums, prunes, avocados, pineapples, eggplant, walnuts and dates and figs are high in compounds known as sero-

tonin precursors or tryptophan and dopamine precursors such as tyrosine. These compounds do not directly generate serotonin or dopamine but make it easier for your brain to manufacture and release these mood-elevating neurotransmitters into your bloodstream. Eating prunes and other dried fruits on a daily basis helps you to stay regular and avoid constipation.

5. Eat organic foods rich in healthy minerals.

Dr. Weil's statement from the conference on Nutrition and Health advocates "counseling consumers that dietary supplements are not substitutes for the whole foods that contain them. They may be useful as insurance against gaps in the diet and as biological therapeutic agents to help prevent or treat specific diseases. Pharmacists, physicians and other health professionals must be educated about their appropriate uses, benefits and dangers." Take these recommendations to your pharmacist and physician.

Increase your intake of essential minerals such as selenium, zinc, calcium, boron, magnesium, iron and copper by eating more fresh fruit, vegetables and seeds and nuts. Incorporate at least one antioxidant supplement (picnogenol, quercitin, ginger, garlic) into your daily diet to reduce the toxicity from dioxins, PCBs and phthalates or other toxic compounds. You'll also want to eat more bioflavinoids—bioactive antioxidants as found in Juice Plus®, and vitamins K, A, C, E, D, ubiquitone or coenzyme Q and folic acid.

Lycopenes are good antioxidants found in watermelon, grapes, tomatoes and some shellfish. Lycopenes are only released by cooking the food. They seem to help to treat dioxin-induced infertility in men. Lycopenes are one class of the 650 carotenoids found in high concentrations in the testicles of normal males and in low levels in infertile males. Experts are studying the use of lycopenes as a nutrient useful in preventing prostate cancer. Current data seems to indicate they do not play a significant role.

6. Do not use plastic containers and plastic wraps for storing food.

The poisons in plastics can leach into the very food you are trying to protect. Be safe and replace plastic with wax paper or glass jars for long-term storage. Only use ceramic or glass dishes for serving or heating food. Never microwave food in plastic containers or bags if you want to avoid dioxin. Even polycarbonate baby bottles and breast pumps, which are supposed to be inert, can contaminate breast milk.

7. Ask your doctor to check your hormone levels.

If you test low in serum or salivary hormones, request a prescription for the deficient hormone. If your doctor won't help you, see an endocrinologist. Remind your doctor to test the free or unbound hormone levels plus the total and protein-bound levels. Saliva tests are only useful for screening for hormone deficiency and are not useful for monitoring of hormone therapy.

Hope is still alive that one day we can clean up our environment and deliver a safe food supply for the American people without the presence of toxins, the EDCs that are destructive to our endocrine system. Until that time, if you want good health you should modify your food choices and focus on a plant-based diet with an intelligent selection of supplements including bioflavinoids, antioxidants and vegetable oils free from trans-fatty acids.

Each person is a powerful force for change. We should all make a noble effort to save this planet for our children. If someone becomes a vegetarian, awareness of this lifestyle choice helps to stop the senseless slaughter of animals. One small change, switching to a plant based diet, can make a difference in stemming the tide of toxic pollution and destruction of our planet! All advances begin with one person, one idea and one goal. Evidence abounds that the foods you eat are not only making you fat but are also exposing you to a high risk of debilitating illness and inability to have babies.

Estrogen and progesterone, although considered female hormones, play an essential role in normal male function just as testosterone does for females. The influence of endocrine disruptive chemicals including the anti-aphrodisiacs—tobacco and alcohol can throw our hormones into disarray. We should all pay attention to the evidence and make life-style changes that will put us in harmony with the ecological forces that make life as a human being so rewarding. Albert Einstein expressed it like this: "Nothing will benefit human health and increase the chances for survival of life on earth as much as the *evolution to a vegetarian diet.*" (Author's italics)

3

HORMONES AND YOUR SEX LIFE

Melatonin, the Hormone of Darkness

Most women and some men have the remarkable ability to fall asleep quickly and wake up promptly and effortlessly. How do they do it? Deep within the recesses of your brain rests the tiny *pineal gland*, home of the remarkable hormone, *melatonin* and the primary timing device and regulator of your body's daily cycles. The pineal gland has been called the body's "third eye" as it connects you with the world of visible light.

The pineal of animals also contains magnetic neurons that are sensitive to the Earth's magnetic field. Roughly the shape and size of a pine nut, the pineal has been the subject of study and speculation through the ages; credited by some for being the body's magical link between the physical and spiritual worlds. A tiny hormone gland that can help you tell the time of day and pinpoint an animal's location in relation to the North Pole sounds pretty amazing.

How does the pineal operate? Twenty-four hours a day, steady as a metronome, specific cells in the hypothalamus move back and forth like the ticking of a built-in clock. When night sets in, as darkness falls, melatonin takes on its sleep-inducing function. Your body is programmed to respond to the darkness by increasing the amount of melatonin. Melatonin reaches its peak between midnight and 2 a.m. when your brain has ten times as much melatonin as it does during the daytime.

How does melatonin compel people to fall asleep at night? The word "melatonin" comes from the Greek word, *melas*, for "black." Melatonin may be your most important hormone since it initiates the process of hormone regulation. The fact that melatonin is switched on by darkness and inhibited by light means that it responds to light directly. When it gets dark, melatonin levels increase. This interplay between melatonin and darkness gives rise to the hormone's title as the "hormone of darkness."

Two opposing systems help induce sleep—the wake-promoting center and the sleep-promoting center. Melatonin activates the sleep-promoting center. While you are asleep, your body is at rest, dreaming and storing up energy for another day of activity. Chemicals called *histamines* activate the wake-promoting center in your brain. In the early morning, daylight enters your eyes, though they are closed, striking the retina and immediately ends up deep within your brain where a timing mechanism kicks in to restore histamine levels to their daytime concentration. Histamine wakes you up as well as making you sneeze and itch.

In the routine day-to-night circadian rhythm, bursts of melatonin pulse into your blood stream every 30 minutes. This rhythmic pattern is so strong that your brain continues to follow the 24-hour cycle even if you cannot perceive light. In other words, this capacity is retained *even for blind people.*

Too much or too little melatonin can disrupt your body's normal response to these daily cycles of light and dark. Maybe you know someone who loves to snack at night or has problems going into a deep sleep. Inadequate levels of melatonin activate such behaviors. In that same manner, too little histamine in the morning creates fogginess and tiredness. This fact becomes especially important when we discuss daytime sleepiness.

Lapses in attention, memory, judgment and just plain fatigue cause automobile accidents, dozing off at the company meeting and accidents on the job. Overworked hospital residents make poor medical decisions due to sleep deprivation. Consistent sleep deprivation will eventually increase the risk for mental and emotional difficulties, poor school performance and accidents

Why is sleep so important? Deep sleep is necessary for creation of memory and the regeneration of neurons within the thinking part of your brain. Specific stages of sleep are involved in forming new memories and even hormones. Deep refreshing sleep is associated with the release of human growth hormone, which helps to regulate your weight and the rate at which you age. Researchers think that the brain is affected adversely by sleep deprivation. When certain patterns of electrical and chemical activity that occur during sleep are interrupted, they delay the brain's ability to function normally. The result... just recall the last time you went without sleep for a single night.

Since melatonin or histamine can change your circadian rhythms, modify your sleep and affect your biologic clock, it should not surprise you to learn that these same chemicals, in the proper balance, can restore your hormonal balance if it goes out of kilter. Melatonin is essential for normal sleep and wake cycles, particularly in the elderly. Yes, as little as *one half of a milligram*, a thousandth of a gram, of melatonin will induce a peaceful sleep in most humans.

The FDA approved a new class of sleeping pill, Rozerem™ (by Takeda), in July of 2005 for insomnia with difficulty initiating sleep. This new medication, prescribed for chronic insomnia, has no withdrawal effects, no addiction and is approved for long-term use but unlike most hypnotics, Rozerem or Ramelteon, is not classified as a controlled substance. Ramelteon works by stimulating a biological brain component, the melatonin receptor, without inducing daytime sleepiness. Rozerem also affects circadian rhythm regulation.

Daytime sleepiness creates numerous problems for many folks: difficulty driving, poor concentration, memory loss and chronic fatigue. Several hormones, especially melatonin, are attuned to normal patterns of light and darkness. Any disruption of these cycles upsets their balance in the body.

What happens when you damage this inner clock that helps you cycle your hormones? Without a functional biological clock, you could not tell the difference between day and night. Disruptions in your circadian rhythms can disturb your entire life cycles. Too much melatonin, for example, can also make people fatigued, confused, depressed and possibly psychotic.

Human beings need balanced hormones plus abundant light to function normally. A lack of adequate lighting can throw our brains into a tizzy. Too much melatonin can aggravate depression or make us feel crazy. Too little histamine generates daytime fatigue. Any disruption of the circadian rhythm of our brains creates imbalance in our hormonal function.

It is for this reason that exposure to high-intensity daylight holds the potential to restore hormonal balance and banish depression from many people's lives. Adding high intensity, full spectrum lighting to every room of your home and workplace promotes restful sleep and helps to eliminate daytime sleepiness. The benefits are unmistakable.

The action of melatonin in the human body is not fully understood, but we know that melatonin levels decrease with age in much the same way as other hormones such as testosterone and growth hormone. These hormones are considered to be age dependent.

Why Do Hormone Deficiencies Lead To Problems?

I often hear from many patients that sleep eludes them at night and if only they could turn off their brains, the way they turn off their computers, they would "sleep like a baby." Actually a baby sleeps most of his babyhood away. The infant's developing brain needs almost 20 hours of sleep in the first year. Lack of sleep brings about irritability, difficulty concentrating and we all know how sleep deprived babies behave.

It's a little different for grown men. They experience a lack of sex drive and increased hunger when they don't sleep well at night. Sometimes, like babies, they get irritable if they don't get their way. Women, on the other hand respond differently to sleep disturbances.

Women come into my office complaining that they have started their menopause and stopped sleeping through the night. They are irritable, constantly in motion and have difficulty concentrating when they don't sleep well at night. They wonder if they need estrogen or progesterone. More often than not the problem is a hormone they seldom think about—melatonin, the sleep hormone.

Like most hormones, melatonin generally follows a predetermined cycle with low concentrations during the day, skyrocketing to ten times that level at midnight. High melatonin levels in the early morning, resulting from reversed daily circadian rhythms can lead to a testosterone deficiency plus sleepiness during the day. Testosterone supplementation can reverse the negative effect of too much melatonin and normalize sleep patterns within three weeks.

Melatonin carries light signals traveling from the pineal gland by a pathway of neurons to the part of the hypothalamus we call the suprachiasmatic nucleus or SCN. This may be a difficult concept to grasp, but please bear with me.

As the timepiece of the brain, the SCN demonstrates both circadian and seasonal fluctuations in vasopressin-expressing cells. What does this mean? In simple terms, by altering the pulses of vasopressin, your anti-diuretic hormone, your biologic clock stop you from waking up to pee during the night. This assures that you have an uninterrupted sleep.

The same system changes with the seasons. Therefore vasopressin is also a light-sensitive hormone. Originating in the SCN, vasopressin, keeps men from urinating during the night or during sexual arousal. Apparently men have greater control in this area than women; loss of control over their bladder function can be a sign that women have lower vasopressin. Oftentimes this "incontinence" is blamed on birth trauma or surgery, but hormone changes can affect women's bladders more than men's.

Tip: If you do waken to go potty during the night, don't turn on the lights or your melatonin levels will be suppressed and you won't be able to get back to sleep.

Since there are sexual differences in the size of the hypothalamus, it becomes obvious that men and women experience light-sensitive hormones in dissimilar ways. In men the size of the cells producing vasopressin is greater than that in women but the neuron cells that secrete oxytocin are the same size. This same segment of brain also determines sexual preference and contains a structure known as the "sexually dimorphic nuclei" or SDN. The SDN of the preoptic area is a tiny area of the hypothalamus, which is two to three times larger in men than in women. It is critical for developing sexual identity and behavior and is extremely sensitive to sex hormones.

Low sex hormones make possible higher blood levels of melatonin during the day and lower levels at night, a reversal of the normal pattern and a factor in many of the symptoms of depression. Lower-than-normal nighttime melatonin promotes wakefulness, stimulates the appetite and disrupts the antidiuretic effects of vasopressin causing frequent urination at night. This results in poor sleep patterns and daytime fatigue.

If you have trouble falling asleep or wake up frequently during the night, then have difficulty getting back to sleep, or wake up too early, you're not alone. According to the National Sleep Foundation's, "Sleep in America" survey, more than half of American adults have sleep problems at least a few nights a week. In fact, insomnia and daytime fatigue are two of America's top health problems and experts have identified lack of sleep as the trigger for many serious disorders ranging from depression to diabetes.

Circadian rhythm disturbances are common in various types of depression. If you've ever been depressed or been close to someone who was, you probably noticed changes in eating and sleeping habits along with moods that swing to the lowest depths. Once something upsets the day-to-night cycle in a depressed person, he or she will have more difficulty functioning normally.

Abnormal sleep patterns are a major symptom in depression, leading to increased weakness, a decrease of sexual drive with an abnormal appetite and daytime sleepiness. The deficiency of melatonin associated with aging results in a reversal of sleep patterns. In spite of the fact that roughly 50 percent of the elderly have trouble sleeping, melatonin levels are rarely measured or supplemented. But it's not only our older citizens who have melatonin imbalances.

When children pass puberty they enter adolescence. Adolescence is the time of the greatest hormonal turmoil. Some hormones rage and others quiver. Sleep cycles are altered in teenagers so that they stay up late and sleep in. They end up with daytime fatigue and no energy for homework or chores. Struggling to get out of bed in the morning can be a warning that depression might develop soon. Sleep difficulties are often associated with depression, weight gain and attention deficit hyperactivity disorder (ADHD).

Pilots and flight attendants who cross several time zones can also become subject to a shortage of certain brain hormones over time. Sometimes these frequent travelers, christened "jet lag junkies," start to feel better at night and on overnight flights. They stay awake the entire night and feel charged and energized the next day. As their sleep needs seem to decrease, they become more tired, with mood shifts at highly inappropriate times. Deep within their brain, the flow of histamine and certain hormones has slowed or stopped.

One study indicates that jet lag from constant travel between time zones can disrupt the melatonin levels creating abnormal sleep cycles leading to memory loss with confusion, internalized anger and psychosis. Low histamine in the brain produces daytime sleepiness, as discussed earlier. This problem is being corrected with a new drug, Provigil®, from Cephalon, which increase brain histamine levels.

Important research on Provigil performed by Leslie Lundt, MD, is discussed in her new book, *Think Like a Psychiatrist*. She writes: "Provigil can help you stay awake and alert. The exact mechanism for Provigil is not fully understood, but it is believed to increase histamine activation in the sleep-promoting area of the brain. There is also evidence suggesting that Provigil works with a dopamine mechanism. Interestingly, the mechanism of Provigil enhances arousal during wakefulness ... but does not interfere with sleep when these neurotransmitters are quiet."

The human body maintains a highly effective self-monitoring balance of hormones through a complex system of regulating factors and feedback loops running from the pituitary to the hypothalamus and modulated by the pineal gland deep within the brain. This balance is maintained by the tight interaction of the neurotransmitters, visible light and hormone regulators. What happens when stress creates an imbalance?

Stress activates the system known as the hypothalamic-pituitary-adrenal or HPA axis, leading to more cortisol (the "stress hormone") circulating through the body. The releasing factor that triggers cortisol is the corticotropin-releasing hormone (CRH). Stress also arouses the nervous system to release quantities of the chemical adrenaline and prepare the body for "fight or flight." Appropriate response to stress is essential for proper performance of tasks and positive social interactions. Exposure of the developing brain to severe or prolonged stress may result in a mental disorder, especially with the passage of time.

Around middle age, degeneration can begin in some neurotransmitter neurons. For example, the normal circadian fluctuations of vasopressin in the brain are diminished in subjects older than 50 years as the number of neurons decreases. Then again, CRH neurons increase in number and are activated during the course of aging. For this reason, your body may respond to stress inappropriately, in a way that may account for hormonal and psychiatric disorders. The severity of these conditions can be negatively affected by your genetics, exposure to harmful environmental factors or the bad timing of stress-producing events in your life.

The most important hormones coping with stress are typically self-regulated by our circadian rhythms, restoring equilibrium much like a crew of computer programmers and repairmen. Signals traveling via the neurotransmitters norepinephrine, dopamine, serotonin and epinephrine help prevent chaos in the coordination of our body defenses during stressful or catastrophic situations.

Do Hormones Create Sexual Arousal?

Anthropologists suggest that nature embeds a constant state of sexual arousal in all humans following puberty in order to assure regular reproduction of our species. The feeling of readiness for sex is merely a reaction to our neurotransmitters. We now understand that many human behaviors may be spontaneously related to interactions between our hormones.

As human beings, we are continually responding to stimulus in our environment. Our resulting actions are known as our behavior. Much of my clinical practice is devoted to the fact that you and I do not have total control over the mechanism of these reactions. As I have already explained, a simple change in our immediate environment, such as a song on the radio, a phone call or a TV movie, sets in motion a series of events including feelings and behaviors that can run the gamut from kissing to sexual intercourse and depressive thinking to food cravings.

One example of the spontaneous response to influences in our environment is the increase in mating behavior in the spring when the weather begins to warm up. A physiologic equivalent would be that in springtime, higher levels of testosterone are released, eliciting amorous feelings that induce courting behavior and "falling in love."

Women often ask me if there is a "loving" hormone because their husbands seem to have lost it. Apparently, the interplay between certain neurochemicals can create feelings of love, triggering a variety of sexually related behaviors. But how can we control these behaviors and how do they differ between animals and humans?

In animals, loving activity includes grooming, mounting and receptive posturing. In humans, love between the sexes prompts a wide variety of dating behaviors and cues. These cues range from receptive body language to signals of intent to seduce. When you fall in love, hormones take over. Difficult as it may be to accept; your emotions and sexual behavior are often due to the circulation of specific hormones and not, as you may have assumed, a direct result of your own needs or desires.

While I would not want to pass judgment on this kind of behavior, it's important that you realize that any factor that adversely influences your endocrine system can make dangerous things happen. Too much testosterone can be as bad as too little.

Alleged "testosterone supremacy" is a misnomer frequently applied to men who are predatory or unkind to women. But the truth is that this kind of behavior has less to do with high testosterone than it does with a badly balanced endocrine system. In other words, stress, negative emotions, gloomy outlook and even aches and pains can be related to low testosterone. Meanwhile, alcohol, street drugs, tobacco and environmental chemicals can create low testosterone and high cortisol.

I am agreeing that "we dangle like puppets on hormonal strings", so eloquently stated by Deborah Blum, in her book, *Sex On The Brain*. She went on to say, "If hormones do profoundly affect behavior, which I believe, though not all do, then they must do so as one of many cast members, not as a solo performer. Our behaviors are, in many ways, wide open to many influences: foods, drugs, injuries, life in all its dimensions." In other words, when we do accomplish activities, hormones are tugging at us in important ways. What happens is not always what you want.

Which hormones are tugging in your relationships? Oxytocin and vasopressin are two hormones that could play critical roles in your arousal and in the establishment of an intimate loving connection, including fathering, mothering and pair bonding. These hormones originate in the hypothalamus, which sits in the center of your brain. The ecstatic hormonal cascade we call "falling in love" involves stimulation of these hormones and others in a complicated process I will try to explain.

Cells in the hypothalamus release vasopressin and oxytocin into your blood circulation. In the fetus, these same hormones play an active role in the birth process. Fetal oxytocin may actually initiate the course of labor and fetal vasopressin plays a role in the adaptation to stress by the newborn. Corticotropin releasing hormone or factor, called CRH or CRF, plays a central role in the stress response of adults by modulating cortisol levels.

Oxytocin is another neurohormone that is heavily involved in your sexual experience. A burst of oxytocin is released at the exact moment of ejaculation. Both sexes experience oxytocin-induced contractions at the moment of orgasm. Women with high oxytocin levels seem to experience multiple orgasms and report greater orgasmic intensity than women with normal levels of this hormone. It thus becomes obvious that your body somehow uses oxytocin for lovemaking.

We might call Pitocin®, a synthetic form of oxytocin, the woman's Viagra. Once prescribed to encourage breast-feeding, Pitocin also increases sexual desire and vaginal lubrication. Why is it only used at the time of delivery to induce contractions?

At the moment of orgasm, these ecstasy-like chemicals or endorphins make us all feel "warm and cuddly." The interplay between hormones and neurotransmitters regulate your sexual life. Pay attention to them, they're important.

What are Neurotransmitters?

Leslie Lundt, author of *Think Like a Psychiatrist*, describes neurotransmitters as follows: "The messengers that deliver messages within the brain are chemicals known as neurotransmitters. We have over sixty neurotransmitters in our brain. Neurons and neurotransmitters are continually assessing the need for more chemical products and, through a complex network of commands and activities; hundreds of powerful drugs emerge in our brain to help keep us functioning at optimal levels. Neurotransmitters are chemical agents that are manufactured by the body from amino acids. They have two primary functions: to *excite* or to *inhibit*. Their role depends on the type of receptor cells at the destination where the message is delivered."

Neurotransmitters such as epinephrine, norepinephrine and serotonin excite your moods, appetite, sleeping, dreaming, energy levels and your perception of pain. Much like the feeling when you narrowly miss a crash on the highway or become angry enough to fight or run away, similar emotions can terrify or motivate you. These responses of your autonomic nervous system are considered *involuntary*, meaning you have no conscious control over them.

Obviously you control many physical acts. Your muscles, for example, move your feet and hands when you will for them to move. We say that these muscles are under your *voluntary* control. By contrast, your body controls many functions without your conscious intervention. We classify these as the Autonomic Nervous System (ANS), which is also known as the automatic nervous system. You might think of the ANS as a self-contained world inside your body with its own brain and systems that run bodily functions without you being aware of its action.

Two systems together comprise the ANS. The background activity of the sympathetic and parasympathetic arrangement, for example, regulates your desire to make love. These systems oppose each other in some ways and support each other in other ways. The sympathetic, as mentioned earlier, excites us when we are fearful or angry. Our pupils dilate, our heart beats faster and our digestive system slows until the problem is resolved. Whenever we feel panic or fear, sudden outpourings of *adrenaline* or epinephrine, discharged from the adrenal gland, stimulate the sympathetic receptors in our nervous system.

The parasympathetic system, in contrast, takes over certain functions when we sense that we are not under attack. The neurotransmitter norepinephrine (NE) regulates most parasympathetic activities. The resulting inhibiting effect produces a slower heart rate, smaller pupils and easier breathing. The NE stimulation of our salivary and digestive glands affects digestion and elimination. The relationship between these chemicals is intimate. Dopamine can be converted into norepinephrine, which becomes epinephrine or adrenaline, as needed. Remember these neurotransmitters for they become more significant as we go on.

A balance between exciting and inhibiting or calming responses is vital to achieve equilibrium and a general feeling of harmony. Sexual arousal in men is a parasympathetic occurrence that can be instantly suppressed by a sympathetic action. In simple language this means that men with an erect penis, prepped for penetration by the effects of sexual arousal, can be blocked by a sensation of panic or anxiety, triggered by adrenaline.

Therefore, relaxation is an important part of successful sexual performance. It is interesting that men and women experience profound differences during sexual arousal. The unconscious, or sympathetic, adrenaline-driven brain dampens arousal in men but stimulates arousal in women. Again you can see the law of opposites attract in action within our own brains.

Women and men are definitely opposite in many ways, attracting each other when it comes to sex but repelling each other when it comes to long-term commitment. Sexual arousal generates increases in concentrations of other hormones such as prolactin, vasopressin, luteinizing hormone (LH) and testosterone. The roles of these hormones are intertwined much like the plots in a soap opera.

Your Sense of Smell and Sexual Attraction

While many animals have a better sense of smell than humans, scent serves us well in finding our mates. Smell registers in a primal part of the brain responsible for memory and emotion. Smell is the only sense that bypasses the rational part of our brains. Why does a man smell "dreamy" or a woman "divine"? These are terms that lovers use to describe their mates. These intangible qualities of those we love are related to sexual attractants triggered by our hormones. It's much like the moth that can follow a solitary molecule that leads it to its mate in a sea of evening aromas.

Like other behaviors we have thought of as fully instinctive, sexual attraction depends on the interactions between hormones and specific neurochemicals named pheromones that affect the "olfactory brain" (our sense of smell). Pheromones are undetectable scents that drive human reproductive behaviors. They are so powerful that merely a few molecules of female pheromones can boost a man's testosterone by up to 150 percent, in seconds. In the same whiff, male pheromones increase testosterone levels in women.

In a single moment, a woman's nose allows her to actually sense the immune system of other humans. Women tend to seek out pheromones characteristic of the immune systems of their fathers. According to Laura Berman, coauthor of the book *For Women Only: A Revolutionary Guide to Overcoming Sexual Dysfunction and Reclaiming Your Sex Life,* which she wrote with her sister, Jennifer, "Women sniff out the best mates via pheromones. It's a concept known as major histocompatability complex, or MHC. The simple explanation is that women unknowingly prefer the scent of men with whom they are best suited to mate, at least immunologically speaking. Basically, the more different a man and woman's immune systems, the better their children's odds are of surviving." Conversely, men prefer pheromones that provide a complementary immune system to their own. These attractions we experience are totally unconscious yet they lead to feelings of sexual arousal.

The hormone responsible for this arousal mechanism is termed the melanocyte stimulating hormone or MSH. This is the same hormone that induces our skin to tan in the presence of sunlight. Complex regulating factors and feedback loops going from the pituitary gland to the hypothalamus and modulated by the adrenal glands above the kidneys maintain a balance of some hormones in the human body. Thus we have a hypothalamic-pituitary-adrenal axis (HPA) much like the love triangles within TV soaps. Each gland affects, attracts and interacts with its target gland within this triangle.

Oxytocin and vasopressin promote feelings of bonding, mutual attractiveness and a highly refined sense of appreciation of the "smell" of your sexual partner. Odors may actually turn us on and off from mates with whom we are reproductively compatible. Next time you think about having sex, take a moment to smell your partner and appreciate the way your brain makes sex such an enjoyable activity while perpetuating the human race. Besides delivering satisfactory sexual performance, hormones allow us to achieve and maintain that sense of well-being that goes along with a life of contentment.

How To Spark Your Sex Life

Hormones are multipurpose. In your brain hormones stimulate your sex organs and ready them for action. Coursing through your body they drive the intense pleasure you feel before, during and after sexual intercourse. And hormones trigger the complex process of creating a firm erection plus the life-long challenge of maintaining that erection during the sex act. "The physiology of erection is like driving a car," according to Arthur Burnett, MD, associate professor of urology at Johns Hopkins. "You can't just turn the key and expect to go anywhere. You also need to hit and hold the accelerator."

A hard penis is a vital component of healthy sexual functioning. Let's take a closer look at what is going on during sexual intercourse—first in a man's body. Since a limp penis cannot penetrate the vagina, the penis must become engorged with blood to complete the sexual act. The process of stiffening the penis for penetration is known as an erection. Following sexual arousal, men develop an erection and women begin to lubricate.

Hormones provide the stimulus to increase the lubrication in a woman's vagina allowing her clitoris to swell in response to contact with a man. Women require quite a bit of foreplay, an average of 20 minutes, to generate these hormones and get their "juices flowing". Both penetration and ejaculation are possible for a man within 30 to 240 seconds. That's not the record, that's simply normal!

Premature loss of an erection is an early sign of sexual dysfunction and possibly heart disease. Women must be on the lookout for these "warning signs" in their sexual partner. An understanding of the factors regulating the human sexual response cycle—desire, arousal, plateau, orgasm and resolution is essential so that you can grasp this concept. The mechanism is almost identical in both sexes and neurotransmitters mediate every one of these five hormonally triggered reactions.

Step 1. Desire
Before a man or woman senses any sexual desire in their body, a sexy image, an evocative smell, a melodious sound or an erotic thought stimulates the brain, creating a state of *sexual arousal*. In the animal world the chemicals that trigger these feelings from scents are known as pheromones. Research indicates that both sexes are stimulated by pheromones. Merchants of perfumes promise better pheromones in a wide array of "love scents", but most of them are of dubious value in seducing a man and yet women eagerly buy them.

Tip: A bit of nervous perspiration is much sexier since your body releases pheromones that can arouse your mate. Bath powder or a quick sponge is a healthy substitute for deodorants if you are in an amorous mood.

Whatever the source of stimulation, our brain immediately senses when we are ready for sexual activity. In the twinkling of an eye, the hypothalamus triggers the release of melanocyte stimulating hormone or MSH, emitting oxytocin and vasopressin.

John Updike in his erotic new novel, *Villages,* provides a less technical but a superb description of desire. He writes, "Sex is a programmed delirium that rolls back death … the black space between the stars given sweet substance in our veins and crevices." Desire is only part of the sexual response but to move up to the next step, it takes more than words, unless you happen to be a poet. Words can turn women on!

The hormone cascade sets off dopamine, triggering the male hormones, testosterone and dihydrotestosterone (DHT). DHT gives rise to the sexual drive while MSH, mentioned earlier, produces arousal. As clarified by psychiatrist Lundt, "Dopamine is a neurotransmitter with a similar effect of boosting moods. It increases a person's ability to concentrate and helps him or her feel motivated to stick to a task." Is sex considered a task? It is for some, though it should always be pleasurable.

Give your dopamine system credit for orchestrating the task your body needs to prepare your sexual organs with lubrication. Dopamine, referred to as the prolactin inhibiting factor or PIF, acts as a neurotransmitter. Therefore it is able to bridge the gap ("synapse") between nerve cells as it sends signals from one neuron to another. The nerve cell receiving the message or the *receptor neuron* sends messages to special dopamine receptors deep inside the brain. These signals activate nerves in the penis that transform it from flaccid to erect. The same signals increase blood congestion and moistness in the vagina.

If the sex act advances perfectly, how does a woman react? A woman's body responds to stimulation from the male hormone testosterone, by the engorgement of her tissues and lubrication of her vagina to encourage receptivity. As a man gets aroused, the "female hormone" estrogen sets up his body for the next step. Estrogen receptors in the male brain, not testosterone receptors, receive messages regarding sexual thoughts required to arouse the penis. In this setting, estrogen receptors are activated by the conversion of testosterone to estrogen in the brain.

It may seem somewhat contradictory but the opposite sex's hormones are what turn on your brain. Estrogen receptors arouse males and testosterone receptors arouse females.

Step 2. Arousal—Clitoral/Penile Erection
Only when that special arousal signal comes from the brain will erection occur. At that exact moment, nerve endings in the penis and the clitoris release a gas, nitric oxide (NO), which allows blood to flow into that organ. Testosterone regulates the amount of nitric oxide release in both sexes. Nitric oxide changes the walls of the blood vessels, swelling arteries so that blood can fill the spongy tissue within the two compartments running along the length of the penile shaft and the clitoris. From an embryologic perspective, the clitoris is really a miniature penis.

As sexual tension increases, muscular tension peaks with heavier breathing, rapid heart rate and rising blood pressure. Women may notice maximal vaginal lubrication and men develop an erection as the penis distends to its maximum capacity. During this step, both sex organs become longer and thicker, often doubling in length from the soft or non-aroused state. Approximately four tablespoons of blood are needed to create an erect penis, about eight times its normal blood volume. Simultaneously, the clitoris doubles its blood supply from one to two teaspoons. The neurotransmitter nitric oxide is intimately involved in this activity in both sexes.

Tiny veins are squeezed shut by the inflow of arterial blood, trapping blood in the penis and keeping it hard until ejaculation occurs. A man cannot urinate while the penis is erect because special vasopressin receptors close off the bladder. This protective mechanism requires the presence of the biologic chemicals: norepinephrine, nitric oxide and adrenaline plus the antidiuretic hormone, vasopressin. Vasopressin and oxytocin are actively involved in promoting the experience, playing a major role in delivering the message that humans are receptive to having sex.

Step 3. Plateau—Ejaculation and Lubrication

During foreplay, a woman's vaginal muscles relax, her clitoris swells and her vagina becomes lubricated. The period of excitation is slower for women, who reach orgasm up to 20 minutes after foreplay while men can usually ejaculate within a minutes of penetration. Timing can easily become mismatched if both partners expect to achieve orgasm at exactly the same time during sexual intercourse.

Triggered by oxytocin from the brain, ejaculation is associated with genital contractions in men and uterine contractions in women. During this step the prostate gland at the base of the bladder, fills up with fluid. This fluid plus secretions from lubricating glands accumulate within the prostate to produce semen, which provides a nutritive liquid, supporting sperm during their frenzied swim toward the egg. Semen is the greater part of the ejaculate.

As the ejaculate, containing millions of tiny sperm, explodes from the penis, the release of oxytocin causes rhythmic contractions of the prostate and the muscles of the pelvis. Oxytocin generates more intense uterine contractions in women, further increasing moisture and lubrication, creating a flushed feeling in the neck, breasts and lips.

Step 4. Orgasm

Sexual climax begins in the groin with an upsurge of sensitivity in the sex organs. Facial contortions, curling of the toes, as a result of spasms of the pelvis, neck, arms and legs, set the stage while sphincters tighten. During orgasm in women, dozens of shudders occur at regular intervals. Just as the timing of the rhythmic twitching of a man's pelvic muscles matches the very same intervals, ejaculate spurts out of the fully erect penis.

Suddenly the message reaches the brain, releasing a gush of neurotransmitters, also triggered by oxytocin. Orgasm occurs both in the brain and in the genitals. When news of this increased sensitivity reaches your consciousness, intense, pleasurable floods of endorphins, dopamine and norepinephrine bathe the deep recesses of your mind. When neurotransmitters engulf the receptors they induce feelings of profound eroticism and euphoria. That's why we find sex so intensely satisfying.

The heightened excitement, overwhelmed by the peaking of subjective pleasure is followed by the release of sexual tension and subsequently the person becomes self-focused as awareness of the sensual experience is diminished.

Step 5. Resolution

After orgasm, a man becomes refractory to sexual stimulation for up to an hour while a woman is ready to orgasm in half that time. Different hormones control these responses. With resolution the body returns to the pre-excitement phase as pelvic congestion is relieved; breathing and heart rate return to normal. In older men, the penis rapidly becomes soft, often within minutes of penetration; in younger men, or with the use of an erection enhancer, a second ejaculation may occur without the loss of erection.

Women can get an extra response, experiencing multiple orgasms that are related to the effects of oxytocin on their hypothalamus and pituitary. Endorphins soothe the brain with a morphine-like calmness, creating an associated "high" feeling. After the male climax, dopamine levels drop and the prolactin hormone kicks in, making it impossible for another erection to take place for one to eight hours. Prolactin acts for only 30 minutes in women, who can achieve orgasm repeatedly, depending on the length and intensity of stimulation or their oxytocin concentration.

Tip: Ask your psychiatrist for a prescription for Pitocin Nasal spray if your sexlife is dead or you do not orgasm!

Why Do Men Lose Interest in Sex?

Many women ask me why their husbands lose interest in sex just about the time they start to enjoy it. I tell them that an energetic and enjoyable sex life is a major ingredient of life satisfaction. Sadly some men cannot enjoy this pleasure because they cannot achieve or maintain a full erection or have a lesser awareness of sexual pleasures. Either hormone imbalance or lack of blood flow is the cause. But men do not share their concerns regarding this or any physical problem with anyone. This may be why men, live shorter lives, suffer more serious diseases and commit suicide more often than women.

If a man starts the day with a firm erection, he feels normal. "Morning wood," as some call early morning erections, is a welcome sign of the normal response of the penis to testosterone. Levels of this hormone usually peak between 6 and 8 in the morning, causing an erection. Because erections take place about the time most men wake up and need to urinate, some men think that this creates the feeling. Not so. Morning erections result from the gradual buildup of testosterone during the night. Even though this is the best time for sexual intercourse, many couples jump out of bed to shower and have breakfast, often ignoring this opportunity to make love. Let me tell you a real story.

Ron, a robust marathon runner and dentist, began having problems with erections at age 58, so he made an appointment with his HMO urologist. He wanted to know if it was normal for a man under 60 to have problems enjoying sex.

"I tested repeatedly with a low testosterone level," he told me. "The clinic took an MRI because they thought there might be a problem in my brain. I think the problem was in their brains. After that I saw a nurse practitioner, who prescribed a series of testosterone injections which hurt and did not help either. Six months later, my testosterone still tested consistently below two hundred." Normal total testosterone levels for adult males range from 300 to 1100 ng/dl or nanograms per deciliter.

At this point Ron was given testosterone skin patches (Androderm®). They just caused itching and he could not tolerate them. When he returned for a follow up, Ron's nurse practitioner had left for a new job and another doctor now suggested he try Viagra and arranged a consultation with an endocrinologist at the same HMO. "This new doctor proceeded to take me back to square one with a lecture on how risky it would be to use replacement hormone therapy, since my levels were not yet zero and how I better be careful and maybe give up on sex, because I couldn't take Viagra. Now I was totally confused, because ten years earlier I had an abnormal EKG, but I had never been on heart medication or treated for any heart problem."

The doctors told Ron he had to take it easy and have sex in a quiet dark room and not get too excited. Maybe he and his wife could do something else. As soon as they showed him his erection-inducing alternatives such as penis injections, he left the clinic.

"My wife and I were extremely frustrated," he reported. "We always enjoyed sex in the morning, when I could do anything and now he was taking away our "special time." You can imagine Ron's disappointment. He wondered if his HMO had treated him fairly or if the treatment the doctor recommended was appropriate. This is a far too familiar story from men in their fifties.

Tip: Try making love in the morning if your husband wakes up with an erection.

As you may already know, two negative characteristics of health maintenance organizations or HMOs are the lack of consistent follow-up and decisions based on cost rather than the benefit to the patient. Skilled medical practitioners, who know that continuity of care is essential, are needed to treat men with erectile dysfunction.

Bouncing a patient from care one provider to another, contradicting previous recommendations without consulting the doctor who made them and regulating medicine according to financial concerns, can work against a patient's best interests. Many generalists are finding traditional medical practices eradicated under the HMO umbrella.

In medical school, doctors are taught the importance of treating hormone deficiencies as vigorously as any disease. That means a diagnosis must be made and the best medicine selected. Viagra is often recommended as a temporary solution for men with erectile dysfunction as if restoring erectile function is a solution to the problem.

Most men don't know they are hormonally deficient until they get tested and the majority doesn't want to discuss it. What do you think happens when your hormone levels start to drop and your hormonal balance goes awry? What does that feel like? Look around you. Mid-life crises are affecting over 40 million people in the US. In spite of what you may have heard, sexual dysfunction does not need to be a consequence of aging. A normal human being should be able to enjoy an active sex life over the entire span of his or her life. Men and women should be able to "do it until they die."

What stops them? Low testosterone is a factor more often than we used to think. Low testosterone, known clinically as hypogonadism, leads to a bulging waist (a potbelly), plus a lack of motivation to get things done. Combine that with low energy and the absence of a sex drive and you have the makings of a disaster.

One of my patients, a 45-year-old lawyer from Kansas, considered dyeing his gray hair and wanted me to check his testosterone levels. His wife said he was just going through a mid-life crisis but he felt that it was more than that. He had lost his desire to lift weights and he needed to use Viagra in order to get a firm erection. When his regular physician refused to check his testosterone, he flew to California to see me and sure enough, his total testosterone was around 164 ng/dl. "What's the problem, Doc?" he asked me. "I don't use drugs, I eat healthy, I go to the gym, why is my testosterone so low?" This is what I told him.

One out of ten men over 40 years of age has hypogonadism, or below normal testosterone levels. Yet medical records show that it is rarely the diagnosis. The interpretation of testosterone levels is so complex that the condition is often overlooked and certainly not treated adequately. Plenty of men and women in their eighties have high normal testosterone—people who are still enjoying sex and looking 10 to 20 years younger than their contemporaries. Alas, this is not the objective most people achieve.

Lack of motivation dampens enthusiasm for hobbies, business ventures and sexual pleasure. Many men think they are just getting old and that there is nothing that can be done to correct the problem of losing their erections.

They couldn't be more mistaken. Just because a doctor tells you that your testosterone levels aren't abnormal doesn't mean that you have to put up with hormone-induced sexual problems. A man can have good sexual function even though tests still show low levels of testosterone. Only when the circulating testosterone falls below minimal levels will erections disappear. At that point hormone supplementation is no longer optional.

The drop in free testosterone usually occurs somewhere in midlife or in the early fifties and can be explained by the general decline of certain hormones during the aging process. Circulating or free testosterone is the form of testosterone you need to remember, as this is the main indicator of sexual ability in both men and women.

When a man has problems with sexual functioning, his wife is far more likely to bring concerns about sexual dysfunction to the doctor than he is. Since this is the role women are taking with their men, they should understand what their husband or partner is going through. This is a common story from men who visit me.

Dale, a rancher from Montana, hates discussing his sexual drive, but after encouragement from his wife decided to write to me. "My sexual drive seems normal," he wrote, "not that I know what normal is. I don't have problems getting erect, maintaining and so forth. I wake up at least once a day with 'morning wood.' I never really paid that much attention to it because I probably only have sex once a week due to my wife's low desire. She suggested I write to you. I usually masturbate two to four times a week. I have felt a decline in sexual desire since my peak, but isn't that normal at age 46?" Again, it was his wife that encouraged him to act.

Dale masturbates more frequently than he has sex with his wife. He blames his wife's lack of sex drive for his declining sexual desire and accepts the idea that familiarity has resulted in boredom in the marriage. Imagine his surprise when he learned that his free testosterone was that of an 80-year-old man. No wonder he was feeling old.

You might expect men past middle age to have some sexual problems but what about younger men? Steve, another patient with erectile dysfunction is an amateur bodybuilder complaining of unusual symptoms. This man was not yet 40 when he began suffering from problems maintaining an erection.

"Doc," he wrote, "perhaps you can steer me in the right direction about keeping my erections. I'm 38 and my sex drive gradually has been diminishing since the age of about 32. Recently it has become much worse. I am unable to have satisfying sex most of the time. I don't have as many morning erections as I use to and if I do they are not strong. My testicles often ache after ejaculation. What can I do? I have seen a doctor although not for ED. My cholesterol is high, but my blood pressure is normal. I don't smoke or drink, I'm not overweight and I have a good relationship with my wife. I do get exhausted easily, and need rest to calm my nerves. I believe I have a sensitive or overactive nervous system."

He was right to pay attention to these physical symptoms, since they are unusual for a man in his thirties. But his self-diagnosis, which might have led to a prescription for tranquilizers, was a big mistake.

As it turned out, Steve's problem was related to his low testosterone level. But if he had simply been given a mood-boosting drug like Prozac or Paxil, his problem could have become more serious. Fortunately, in his case, a simple test led to a correct diagnosis and testosterone replacement therapy. His question was answered. It's important to realize that not every patient with Steve's symptoms suffers from low testosterone. But it is important for doctors to check hormone levels in patients, like Steve, before recommending a course of treatment.

Silence creates a difficulty in diagnosis for both doctors and their patients. Doctors depend on patients to tell them what is wrong yet they seldom ask about their sexual performance. Men are not alone in keeping their sexual problems secret. Most women are more candid with their hairdressers than they are with their gynecologists. I find that women try to discuss sexual problems with other women but seldom with their husbands and rarely with a physician.

Young adults and teenagers, the highest risk group for sexually transmitted disease, hardly ever discuss sexual problems with their doctors. Teenagers prefer to discuss sex with friends who aren't trained in these matters. They usually end up bragging and exaggerating instead of telling the truth. Doctors know that men are especially reluctant to talk about their sexual problems and should take the initiative to discuss this subject with their patients or their partners.

Erectile Dysfunction and What to Do About It

Erectile dysfunction is due to inadequate blood volume filling up the spongy penile tissues. A non-erect penis contains about eight cubic centimeters of blood compared to a fully erect penis engorged with 62 cubic centimeters of blood. That's eight times the normal volume of penile blood! For most men ED (erectile dysfunction) refers to "inadequate" erections, meaning they are unable to achieve or maintain an erection sufficient for satisfactory sexual performance. Some men think they have ED if their morning erections are weak or disappear. They're both right!

Erectile function is dependent on the penis receiving its full dose of blood on a daily basis. An inadequate release of the gas, nitric oxide prevents the blood vessels in the penis from filling with blood, resulting in anything from an impaired erection to complete impotence. If for some reason, erections do not develop during the night while the man is in REM or deep sleep, then eventually these tissues will scar and shrink, causing erectile dysfunction. The penis needs to become filled with blood on a daily basis in order to avoid scarring. The saying, "If you don't use it, you'll lose it" is definitely true in this case!

Any process that decreases blood volume to the penis or does not keep the blood within the penis will obviously result in unsatisfactory erections. Men with ED, triggered by a hormone disorder, should be treated appropriately, first with hormone replacement, followed by erection enhancers such as Viagra®, (Pfizer), Cialis® (Lilly/ICOS) and Levitra® (Bayer). Every so often dopamine stimulants, for example the antidepressant bupropion (Wellbutrin® from Glaxo Smith-Kline), are also needed.

Viagra® (or sildenafil), the first erection enhancer, was developed in recognition of nitric oxide's crucial role in causing an erection. The chemical effect of sildenafil was discovered by accident as a way to increase the amount of nitric oxide in the penis. The little blue pill in doses of 25 to 100 milligrams, taken as needed, is an effective treatment with few side effects, for men suffering from erectile dysfunction.

The causes of ED range from the effects of certain drugs to depression and psychological impotence. The use of certain antidepressants can stop normal sexual function once they suppress oxytocin activity. Discontinuing the medication will reverse this effect. With each year men age, the risk of ED increases by 10 percent. ED is associated with changes in liver function, diabetes, obesity, drug and alcohol abuse, zinc deficiency, over-the-counter medications, heart disease, lower urinary tract symptoms, heavy smoking and depression. Eliminating or correcting any of these issues can improve ED.

A current study using low dose Viagra, 10 mg., along with low doses of testosterone of 25 mg. per week or 50 mg. every two weeks, investigates a unique concept. The majority of healthy men over the age of 65, reported "significant improvement in erectile function and this improvement lasted for more than two years," according to Dr. Fredrick Ellyn at the Chicago Medical School. No side effects were seen with this regimen. These were normal men without any complaint of ED.

When the reason for ED is unknown, Viagra, Levitra or Cialis are often highly effective. They increase the response of the penis to sexual stimulation by enhancing the amount of nitric oxide in the organ. Viagra cannot produce a libido. Viagra doesn't work unless there is already enough testosterone on board for sexual desire. Viagra has no effect in the company of a non-existent sexual drive!

Libido is an instinctual, creative emotion. The loss of libido is one of the first signs of a potential sexual problem. The dictionary defines libido as "the instinctual craving or drive behind all human activities." Sigmund Freud said, "Libido is the energy all animals have to fulfill the goals of their lives." We almost always think of libido in sexual terms. "My libido is low," grumbles many a menopausal woman or elderly man, meaning sex has lost its appeal.

Lawrence Hakims, chief urologist at the Cleveland Clinic, points out in his book, *The Couple's Disease,* that about 13 percent of the 30 million men affected with sexual dysfunction are treated, but less than five percent of those affected with a loss of libido actually seek help. These figures are shocking when you realize that sex is one of the great pleasures in life. Hormones definitely play a role in creating your libido. They regulate how energetic you feel as you tackle the challenges you face from day to day, including the success of a good sexual experience. It's important to pay attention when your mate loses his or her motivation for lovemaking.

Impotence, the most common sexual disorder, refers to the total inability to get an erection. The risk of this condition increases in men as they age, but three out of four men are too embarrassed to discuss their sexual concerns with their doctor. This is nonsense. The doctor isn't going to point a finger of blame at the patient. Psychological weakness is highly unlikely to be the basis for this problem. In the vast majority of cases, more than 85 percent of the time, the cause is a physical problem.

Still, if there is an emotional component, getting professional advice is the quickest way to restore normal functioning. Wives should take a proactive role in this condition. I think a major reason for the gap between what we need and what we seek is that we don't take the time to sit quietly and sense our bodies.

Does Viagra Work for Everybody?

Though we know a lot about sexual urges that are driven by our hormones, sexual problems are still far too common in our society. One out of three American men and three out of four women has some degree of sexual dysfunction. Viagra-like erection enhancers are often advertised as the best solution for sexual dysfunction, but the plain fact is that these drugs cannot generate the human sex drive.

The world of male sexual performance changed forever in March of 1998 when the Food and Drug Administration (FDA) approved the prescription sale of Viagra by Pfizer Pharmaceuticals. The drug made history as the first medicine that would enable a man to achieve an erection and maintain it throughout the act of sexual intercourse. Viagra has freed millions of men in more than 90 countries from the disappointment of ED (erectile dysfunction). Worldwide, sales of the drug exceed a billion dollars per year.

From the jokes and comments made about Viagra, you would think it's a magic pill that brings sexual fulfillment to all men. Viagra has become a household word associated with sexual arousal. Pop Viagra in your mouth and enjoy blissful sex.

Pfizer makes no such claims about its popular drug, warning men who take it that a dose of Viagra will not enhance sexual desire. Without sexual stimulation, a man who has taken Viagra, as prescribed, will feel no effect except a flushed face.

As an erection-enhancing drug, Viagra succeeds in about 70 percent of men who try it. Due to the high demand for the drug, Viagra is prescribed for men complaining of sexual difficulties before their testosterone levels are measured. Normal men, who grumble that they do not respond sexually the way they did in the past, should have their hormone levels checked first. Regrettably, in today's society, the focus is usually on function and not feeling.

While making it possible for men with sexual dysfunction to experience an erection, Viagra also provides a hidden benefit. The drug cuts recovery time *in half* following sexual intercourse. A firm erection with a shortened recovery time—no wonder Viagra is so popular! Viagra also gives men enough time to give their wives an orgasm.

Then again, giving a man an erection enhancer is not the answer to restoring his virility. Men need sexual arousal in their brain for their penis to become hard regardless of their Viagra dose. Yet the effects of Viagra are so powerful that some men use it before each sexual encounter. The right hormonal balance and an ideal amount of testosterone or estrogen are essential for normal sexual function.

For almost two thousand years, the underlying mechanisms that make erection possible have eluded us. At long last experts have developed science-based assumptions that explain both the neurological and physiological characteristics of the erection. New drugs have appeared on the market to compete with Viagra, promising to deliver an erect penis faster with fewer side effects. Two of these new erection-enabling drugs are Cialis and Levitra. Cialis lasts four times as long as Viagra and is taking over market share.

Unfortunately, most men associate erections with sex drive and view their ability to get erections as a sign of their sexual prowess. Medically speaking, they are wrong. Researchers have found that men can achieve an erection chemically without any sexual drive or arousal whatsoever. Do you remember that autonomic nervous system and its two components?

Drugs that block the activity of the sympathetic nervous system can be injected directly into the penis, (Ouch!) permitting an erection to occur. But nitric oxide (NO) must be present. This vital gas, produced within our arteries, causes the vessel walls to relax, once sexual arousal has been achieved. Medications like Viagra can induce an erection in men with a less-than-normal sexual drive, but the effect is mainly the result of nitric oxide release in the blood vessels of the penis.

Not everything about Viagra is wonderful. Men who depend on Viagra regularly to maintain erections can become psychologically dependent or impotent without it. As I mentioned, Viagra is merely an erection enhancer. Again, without adequate testosterone, Viagra has no effect.

Viagra has been tried in women with female sexual arousal disorder. The use of Viagra for women is an off-label use and if the hormones of these women were to be studied, I suspect we would find that what these women really need is testosterone.

Testosterone (T) is, I believe, a far more effective stimulant of the sex drive in women or men than Viagra. Testosterone is essential for a full firm response in the erect penis, according to studies by André Guay, professor of Endocrinology at the Center for Sexual Function, the Lahey Clinic at Harvard. Dr Guay is the researcher who just published the latest normal T ranges in older men.

Studies in Germany indicate that during sexual excitement, levels of testosterone increase time and again in the penis itself and those men with ED had levels that were 27 percent lower than in normal men. Dr. Guay's research showed that raising testosterone had a positive effect on sexual function but as T levels decreased so did the response to Viagra. For men, testosterone is vital in achieving an erection. A man with low T may develop a strong erection with the assistance of Viagra, but without sexual arousal, nothing much will happen once his penis becomes firm. It takes testosterone to rouse a man's sex drive to complete the sexual act. The same hormone stimulates a woman's drive as well.

Patients who tried Viagra and did not like the results are rare, but Todd is one man who took Viagra twice and decided it was not for him. "I would not take this medicine again," said Todd, a tall Texan. "My reaction was a bad headache with sinus pressure and a warm sensation in my ears." He was disappointed with Viagra's effect on his erection. "With manual stimulation after taking Viagra I became erect," he said, "but without continual stimulation my erection immediately started to go down. I was not able to achieve orgasm through intercourse though I remained hard and when I finally reached orgasm with manual and oral stimulation it felt like nothing at all."

Todd said sorrowfully, "I was unable to achieve orgasm through vaginal intercourse. The erection from Viagra lasted for over an hour until I was exhausted and no longer interested in continuing because of the lack of sensation, or my partner had enough."

Todd would probably be much happier using testosterone supplementation to help improve his erections but the combination of testosterone and Viagra could provide an optimal sexual experience. Unlike Todd, many men who are impotent find a whole new outlook on life with Viagra. Their sexual performance improves to such a degree that they are willing to put up with the relatively minor side effects. Viagra has brought sex out of the closet and has all but replaced the use of injectable prostaglandins, once used to induce firm erections.

One reason for Viagra's popularity is the fact that, Americans like taking pills a lot better than using creams, patches, or injections. The penile prostaglandin insert (Muse® by Vivus) was the least popular of all types of treatment designed to enhance the sexual experience, even though it worked 85 percent of the time. Another factor in the success of Pfizer's Viagra is the large number of men who have some degree of sexual dysfunction and are willing to try a pill to solve their problem. But there's something even better than Viagra.

A Safe Aphrodisiac for Men and Women

The word "aphrodisiac" comes from the name, Aphrodite, the goddess of love and beauty in Greek mythology and means "arousing or increasing sexual desire or potency." From jasmine to onions, from Yohimbine to Spanish Fly, sex-enhancing substances have been popular throughout the ages. Ancient documents tell us that aphrodisiacs are as old as civilization and as varied as human nature. Aristotle mentioned Cantharides, a powder made from dried blister beetles and applied to the penis to irritate and stimulate it to action. The mandrake, a plant from the potato family, has been used as a sexual stimulant since Old Testament days. Some attempts at heightening sexual pleasure border on the bizarre such as the habit of a Chinese emperor who is said to have kept a herd of deer so he could drink their blood to increase his sexual prowess.

If you want more love making in your sex and are looking for a way to add spice to your sex life, consider the benefits of testosterone therapy. It's a lot easier than herding reindeer or collecting beetles. This hormone is a wonder drug that can give you or your spouse more energy and a sense of well-being as it reduces your body fat while increasing your muscle mass. Of course, whether you are a man or a woman, you still have to exercise and watch your calories. As part of a hormone replacement therapy program (HRT) prescribed by your doctor, testosterone is also good for your heart and might prevent heart disease.

Unlike Viagra, testosterone can restore erections within 24 hours of administration without any sexual stimulation. As a matter of fact, the frequency of erections during the day is primarily a testosterone function. Testosterone is safe for men with heart disease; regardless of the medication they use and has a 60-year track record of medical safety in both sexes. By contrast, Viagra is simply a treatment for erection difficulties in men without heart problems.

Tip: If your doctor reaches for a prescription for Viagra, Levitra or Cialis without doing a blood test, get a second opinion.

Like most people, you'd love to be able to enjoy sex more often, but before you can have great sex, the sex hormones in your brain must be working properly. The essential hormone that makes it possible for you to experience a potent sexual desire is testosterone. Testosterone is your body's true aphrodisiac. This hormone stimulates sexual desire in either sex without irritation or dangerous side effects.

The ability of testosterone to improve sexual craving was first noted in the early 1940s. As the years rolled by, more evidence accumulated regarding the multiple benefits of testosterone therapy. In 2001, Malcolm Carruthers, MD, a British physician, noted in his book, *The Testosterone Revolution*, those men with higher free testosterone possess a superior degree of business motivation in addition to a more robust sex drive than do professionals with less testosterone in their systems. Among his London patients, Dr. Carruthers found that actors and prosecuting attorneys had the highest testosterone levels and the strongest drive. The increased ambition to succeed in business, stimulated by testosterone, seemed to ensure superior function in both the boardroom and the bedroom.

"Hmm," you may be thinking, "Dr. Kryger really believes in testosterone therapy for a happy sexual life." You are absolutely correct! Of all the hormones circulating in our bodies, I do believe testosterone has the greatest potential for helping men enjoy a more vibrant sex life and reap other benefits in the process. You will witness my enthusiasm for this hormone throughout this book.

In my clinic we encourage my patients to have their hormone levels tested as part of their annual exam. That way, as soon as problems arise, we can determine if hormonal deficiencies could be part of the solution.

Is it possible to find out your own testosterone levels? Yes! Testosterone and other hormones can be easily measured in saliva. Nevertheless, accurate determination of a subnormal testosterone or cortisol may require more than one test. Saliva, a secretion of the salivary glands, contains only the free or circulating hormones and can therefore be used as a highly effective screening test. A low reading of free salivary testosterone indicates that a person may be suffering from inadequate testosterone.

Knowing your total testosterone levels will not always predict your sexual function or give your doctor a complete hormone profile. Saliva tests measure the tiny quantity of free testosterone, about one to four percent of the total testosterone that circulates in the blood stream of men. The rest is bound to proteins and is maintained as a storage form of testosterone.

Restoring testosterone to levels that are normal or slightly above normal can be beneficial for men and women alike. An above-normal level gives a person an opportunity to feel what it's like to have the testosterone of a younger person. Studies at Johns Hopkins Medical Center, investigating the use of testosterone supplementation in men with normal hormone levels, found no harm resulting from higher testosterone capacity for a short period of time.

Low testosterone should always be interpreted in the context of symptoms and not by numbers alone. While some men can have totally normal sexual function with very low levels of testosterone, others lose their erectile function when levels are in the normal range. The normal range for serum total testosterone varies by as much as 400 percent at different ages in a man's life. The same is true for women. Some women prefer higher testosterone levels in order to feel vibrant and alive! Men need to pay special attention to their body's hormone levels, due to the teeter-totter relationship between many hormones, keeping in mind that low testosterone levels are associated with higher-than-normal estrogen levels. Estrogen is important in men for their usual sexual aggression.

Men who are low in estrogen may notice impairment in word-finding ability plus a lack of nipple sensitivity, low sexual aggression and testicular shrinkage. Women with low estrogen notice a decline in memory and reaction time. Another important mechanism in the interplay of sexual hormones is the conversion of free testosterone to DHT in the brain.

This fact is significant in understanding the action of the male hormone. Dihydrotestosterone (DHT) is considered to be a powerful form of testosterone as it regulates sexual libido in both sexes promoting sexual arousal and erectile function. DHT is the same hormone that actually causes adolescents to develop beard and body hair, a deeper voice and enlarged genitals—traits we call *secondary sexual characteristics*. This process is genetically controlled and is an innate part of growing up for boys.

Men probably have low DHT levels for one of two reasons: they don't make enough of the enzyme that converts testosterone to DHT, or else some factor is blocking its activity. Tests to measure DHT levels are still in the experimental stages as this book is being prepared for printing and two slightly varied forms of DHT have been recently identified. Since the information about DHT is so new, doctors seldom consider DHT in their evaluation of sexual dysfunction.

The patient and the doctor may agree that their sexual dysfunction is worsened by a hormonal deficiency, but the return to a normal sex life is not always an easy one. I am constantly amazed at what some patients go through to get help for an obvious testosterone deficiency.

Melinda, a 50-year-old housewife came to see me about her 56 year-old husband Jason, who had been receiving testosterone injections from their family doctor. When he was only 47 years old, Jason experienced complete erectile dysfunction and was found to have very low testosterone levels of 130 ng/dl, (250 to 900 ng/dl is normal for his age group). Jason's doctor gave him monthly injections of testosterone, but they seemed to work for only ten days. The couple moved several times and every time he switched doctors, he received the same prescription.

"We think that the amount he is currently getting is far less than originally prescribed because they have no effect at all, when used in conjunction with Viagra," Meribeth told me (notice once again the wife is acting as the husband's patient advocate). "We feel this has been a waste of time and money." She went on to say that Jason's current physician wouldn't increase the dose. "He says it can cause prostate cancer," she said. "We went through another disruption in his treatment for over six months when he didn't receive any injections because the drug was unavailable."

After triple bypass surgery, Jason was placed on Lipitor®. He complained of pain in his muscles and the dosage was cut in half. Now Jason's wife was getting desperate, wondering if his problem with Lipitor is related to the lack of testosterone in his body. He has all the symptoms of low testosterone levels. Where could she go to find real help for her husband?

Melinda is not alone in her futile search for a doctor who will deal knowledgeably with her husband's problems. Too many doctors are turning a deaf ear to their patients. Why? Some are not comfortable prescribing hormones for men. Others just need to "listen" carefully to the evidence showing how beneficial an adequate testosterone therapy program can work for men like Jason.

Until the start of the new century, the standard of care for testosterone replacement has been the use of injections of synthetic esters of testosterone. The treatment showed immediate and impressive results. A single testosterone injection generated a temporary feeling of well-being, greater strength and the return of sexual desire. Unfortunately, these benefits were short-lived. An injection may deliver a high dose of testosterone at first but then the level subsides over several days. The potential side effects from the fluctuations and liver conversion included: hair loss, liver damage, unstable moods, abnormal cholesterol and terrible acne.

The injection of synthetic testosterone can also result in enlargement of the prostate, an accelerated progression of a hidden or undiagnosed prostate cancer, increased thickening of the blood from too many red blood cells and a variety of psychological changes. In older men, several problems are associated with testosterone administration by injection into the large muscles of the body.

So, though testosterone injections represent one of the older and cheaper techniques for delivering the hormone, today the preferred delivery system for testosterone is the use of testosterone preparations applied directly to the skin as patches, creams and gels. These methods work well and produce fewer side effects than injections or implants of testosterone pellets under the skin.

In their search for more innovative dispensing systems for testosterone, Columbia Laboratories received FDA approval in 2003 for a new topical medication named Striant™. Striant delivers testosterone from "oral" patches shaped like tablets that are stuck under the upper lip. Unfortunately, Striant releases testosterone for only 12 hours and so it must be applied twice a day. This method has not found much popularity except for men, who are divers or swimmers and are in the water all the time.

Topical Testosterone Therapy

When testosterone was first synthesized, it was used to treat a common heart complaint termed angina—a pressing pain in the central chest induced by low oxygen levels delivered to the heart. In a more recent study in Great Britain, men with angina reported less pain after applying a low dose of topical testosterone. Topical simply means that the hormone is applied directly to the skin. This was a *single blind*, placebo study, in which the men did not know what they were using but the doctors were aware of the therapy.

The Latin word, "placebo" means, "I shall please." The term, "the placebo effect," refers to the ability of neutral substances to create positive feelings once the person taking them believes they are all-powerful. Scientists estimate that the placebo effect brings about over 40 percent of the results observed with many drugs. In a clinical placebo controlled study, one group being tested receives a neutral substance or placebo while the other gets the substance being studied. The majority of the patients taking testosterone in this study experienced less pain and improved blood flow to the heart as compared to the placebo group. In these clinical trials, the testosterone was applied directly to the skin and absorbed directly into the blood stream via a method called *transdermal delivery*.

Topical testosterone is a relative newcomer to the field of hormone replacement therapy. It has been widely observed that men using the topical testosterone preparation report a remarkable feeling of well-being. Not surprisingly, several new topical testosterone products were approved for the U.S. market since the new millennium. This is not exactly breakthrough science, for in Europe transdermal hormone creams and gels have been used for over ten years.

Although the FDA does not approve them for marketing to the public, pharmacists who are able to prepare topical or transdermal products such as these are identified as "compounding pharmacists." They follow techniques for mixing bioidentical hormones with chemicals that enhance their absorption through the skin, a new and effective form of hormone distribution. For many years, compounding pharmacists across the country have been preparing these products as prescribed by a doctor. The FDA allows compounding pharmacists to fill a prescription for *any type of FDA-approved product* used for the doctor's own patients.

Hormone preparations compounded for transdermal use provide a relatively inexpensive solution to the side effects reported with oral or injectable hormones. Women with sexual dysfunction have also been treated successfully with testosterone in a compounded cream form as an alternate strategy for treating their loss of sexual pleasure. Psychiatrist Susan Raiko states in her book, *The Hormone of Desire,* that the addition of a pea-sized amount of topical testosterone cream applied to the mucous membrane of the genitals effectively saturates the local skin receptors with testosterone. For some women, applying the testosterone directly to the clitoris, the female equivalent of the male penis, enhanced sexual sensation. This is not an accepted standard of testosterone therapy.

Today treatments with topical testosterone gels have entered mainstream medicine. Doctors finally recognize that inadequate hormone levels disrupt essential sexual outcomes such as vaginal lubrication in women, erectile function in men and sexual interest in both. For a successful outcome, a trained physician who supervises the course of treatment must monitor dosage requirements.

With the release of the latest testosterone gel, Testim® by Auxillium in 2003, options for safe treatment with low potency testosterone expanded. No man or woman lacking an adequate supply of this vital hormone should be denied the benefits and the restoration of their normal sexual vigor. To date, a testosterone product for women has not been released.

Tip: If you are a woman experiencing loss of libido, your physician can ask any compounding pharmacist to prepare a 0.5% testosterone cream for a short trial.

How Does Estrogen Affect Male Sexual Function?

Estrogen is so closely linked in our minds to feminine qualities that you may be surprised to learn that it is essential for men's sexual function as well. As important as "the female hormone" is to women, estrogen plays a vital role in the body chemistry of men. Men manufacture only small amounts of estrogen in their testicles, but that's enough to help create a healthy libido, support sperm production, protect hair and skin and strengthen their bones. As we have already discussed, men who are low in estrogen notice a lack of nipple sensitivity or experience testicular shrinking. On the other hand, women with low estrogen notice a decline in memory, reaction time and hot flashes.

As one of the most powerful hormones in the human body, estrogen generates an extensive collection of consequence in women. It stimulates the ovaries to produce mature eggs; signals the endometrium—the lining of the uterus, to grow in preparation for a fertilized egg. Estrogen acts upon many other parts of the body including: the brain, breasts, kidneys, liver, blood vessels and bones. Moreover estrogen regulates the appropriate functioning of additional hormones.

Estrogen is not a single hormone but a trio of hormones, working together to perform a complex network of tasks. We have already spent some time discussing estradiol or E2, the most biologically active of these three hormones. The other two are estrone and estriol. In a healthy young adult female, the typical mix of these hormones is 10 to 20 percent estrone, 10 to 20 percent estradiol and 60 to 80 percent estriol. This ratio is not accidental. Mother Nature sorted through the possibilities over the millennia and came up with this optimal hormonal balance for women. The three estrogen types together are basically the "*conjugated estrogens.*"

Estrogen is essential for normal sexuality, but it can become a dangerous complex if its levels get too high. The link between estradiol (E2) and breast cancer is well documented, although some medical researchers believe that if high levels are experienced over a long period of time, *either* estradiol or estrone can lead to a higher risk of breast cancer. Furthermore, an excess of E2 has been shown to *decrease* the action of either testosterone or DHT. When tested in other mammals, estrogen has also been implicated in causing endometriosis and sex organ cancers in both sexes.

In women, an estrogen deficiency can result in the loss of sexual thoughts, vaginal dryness, memory loss and feelings that someone turned up their thermostat. To counter these negative results, one out of five postmenopausal women uses some type of E2/estrogen supplement as part of her postmenopausal hormone therapy.

Close monitoring is essential if women make use of an estrogen supplement alone, without progesterone. Every two years, regular PAP smears and breast exams with mammography with ultrasound or thermography are suggested. The newer techniques are more sensitive in detecting breast lumps.

Testosterone produces some of its results through the production of estrogen. In fact, testosterone is the primary source of estradiol in your body. Created by the interaction of enzymes and cells in our sex organs, testosterone is made in the testicles of men and the ovaries of women. However, the aromatase enzyme complex, responsible for this conversion, is found throughout the body and the brain.

It is surprising to learn that the average 60 year-old male has more circulating estrogen in his bloodstream than the average 60 year-old female. Although estrogen might have numerous beneficial effects for menopausal women, excess amounts of E2 may be catastrophic for men.

Athletes who use testosterone to beef up their physical prowess don't want any of their testosterone diverted to estrogen. They want the maximum benefit from their supplements, so they self-medicate with anti-aromatase drugs that interfere with the formation of estradiol. This is not a good idea since these drugs diminish sexual arousal and may increase memory loss.

Estrogen has both good and bad effects. On the positive side, estradiol improves memory by stimulating nerve cell growth and survival in the brain. This reaction was once believed to delay the onset of senility and memory loss, such as observed with Alzheimer's. Estrogen is supposed to keep your skin and hair soft and checks balding in men. The negative effects of E2 include activation of cancer cells and worsening of autoimmune diseases such as rheumatoid arthritis or the more rare conditions of Lupus, Scleroderma or Sjogren's syndrome.

As men grow older, estradiol levels tend to stay more or less constant but their testosterone levels drop. The resulting change in the ratio between testosterone and estradiol can cause an apparent excess of the "active" estrogen. Eugene Shippen discusses this phenomenon he calls "estrogen dominance" in his book, *The Testosterone Syndrome.* He believes that estradiol is actually the "primary active estrogen in all women." Furthermore estrogen can act as an *anti-androgen*, working in opposition to male hormones and interfering with the beneficial effects of testosterone.

The relationship between testosterone and estrogen is universal in other animals as well as humans. When testosterone goes up, estrogen usually goes down and vice versa. Too much estrogen can be extremely harmful. Excess estrogen among men is so prevalent today that the E2 levels of men age 54 are higher than those of the average woman at age 59. It's one of the ironies of endocrinology that while women are taking estrogen supplements, excessive estrogen plagues men.

As John F. Kennedy once said in another context, "life isn't fair."

How is Sexual Function Affected by Prolactin?

Pigs and some other animals can prolong intercourse for hours after ejaculation. What stops humans from ejaculating repeatedly? The answer is prolactin, another hormone from the pituitary gland. Prolactin is also responsible for the suckling reflex. When an infant nurses at its mother's breast, prolactin is secreted, allowing a woman to eject milk from her breast.

Nursing women have increased levels of prolactin, ("pro," meaning "for the purpose of" and "lactic" for "milk"). The production of prolactin brings in the breast milk and works to preclude another pregnancy from happening right away. In this same way prolactin causes women to feel less sexual desire after giving birth. In addition, as dopamine levels drop following ejaculation, prolactin increases in order to bring about the refractory period preventing another erection from taking place. Prolactin inhibits sexual desire, permitting breast-feeding to act as a type of birth control for the mother during the first year of a baby's life.

In women, abnormally high levels of prolactin have been associated with the termination of their menstrual period, infertility and decreased sexual activity. In men, prolactin has been considered detrimental to sexual function. When estrogen rises, so does prolactin, working to impair testosterone secretion and its triggering control mechanism, luteinizing hormone (LH). High prolactin can lead to a total loss of libido, with consequences that can be devastating or at least embarrassing.

Scientists have found that prolactin creates the refractory period after ejaculation. Without this mandatory period of sexual inactivity, men could not rest adequately after orgasm to recover in time for their next sexual encounter. Erectile dysfunction has been described in men with abnormally high—and unusually low—levels of prolactin. This suggests that there is more to prolactin than the simple blocking of uninterrupted erections. At one time, too much prolactin, from the presence of a prolactin-secreting brain tumor was thought to be a rare cause of male sexual dysfunction. Brain scans were often used to aid in the diagnosis. For many years if a man complained about his sexual drive, the idea was that there must be something wrong with his brain. Some doctors and some wives still think this way today.

With all the stages required for the sequence that is necessary for a man and a woman to enjoy mutually satisfying sex, it's amazing that it even happens, but thanks to the aphrodisiac effects of DHT, with or without Viagra or the beneficial effects of light on the human species, we will continue to evolve and procreate the planet.

In review, the three sex hormones: progesterone, DHT and estrogen interact with oxytocin, prolactin and human growth hormone to modify the release of testosterone into our bloodstream. Testosterone both increases melatonin and decreases cortisol levels. Prolactin escalates during stress when cortisol levels are at their highest and dopamine levels are fading, leading researchers to conclude that stress could be the major reason for sexual dysfunction. Oxytocin and growth hormone both suppress prolactin, which can completely halt testosterone's action on the penis. This convoluted endocrine masterpiece allows your body to fine-tune itself. At the same time, this interplay of hormones brings about various sexual behaviors, involving our senses that communicate via chemical neurotransmitters. The 36 hormones that operate your endocrine system have something important to say about how you can help them work for your ultimate happiness.

4

HORMONES AND YOUR HAPPINESS

What Is the SAD Disease?

By now you may realize that humans and animals depend on light for health and normal development. Problems surface when the interrelationship between hormones and visible light is disrupted. Scientists have given names to these light disorders. In Scandinavian countries low light levels cause "winter blues" or Seasonal Affective Disorder (SAD). Seasonal mental disorders occur in many parts of North America and northern Europe when the intensity of the sun decreases in wintertime.

Seasonal Affective Disorder results from a pineal gland that is not functioning properly. People with SAD face depression each autumn or winter because it is a cyclical disorder such as those we discussed previously. For victims of SAD, the darkness of winter brings sleepiness, adds pounds and heightens cravings for carbohydrates. They become unhappy, gain weight and sleep too much. If this describes you or your guy, a nonmedical solution is available.

The further you live from the equator, the more likely you are to suffer from SAD. People living in Scandinavia and in the northern latitudes of the US and Canada have the highest rates of this mood disorder. High solar light areas around the equator where you can travel to escape SAD, include such vacation spots as the tropics of Africa, the Caribbean, Mexico, Israel, Australia and the South Pacific. In these locations you can enjoy real light year round, which protects your brain from SAD. These are great places to visit during the winter to help keep your hormones in balance, especially if you suffer from SAD.

A long trip to a sun-drenched vacation site is not the only way to correct Seasonal Affective Disorder. A new drug, approved a short time ago for treating jet lag and shift workers, called Provigil® (or modafinil, by Cephalon) stimulates brain histamine. This and another novel drug (Norvigil®) will help people cope with the long dark sleepless nights that can lead to symptoms of depression. Light therapy, a novel treatment for SAD, will be discussed later in this chapter.

Anhedonia—the Absence of Happiness

Steve, once an avid golfer has a lean muscular body and holds down an executive position at a major financial services company. His career is secure, his family intact, his wife accommodating, his home comfortable, but Steve seems incapable of enjoying his good fortune. At the office he goes through the motions and barely covers the details. At the end of the day, he goes home feeling tired and sad. He doesn't eat much, goes to bed early and says almost nothing to his wife, Melanie, or five year-old daughter. Is he just bored or is Steve severely depressed?

Loss of interest in hobbies and isolation from friends and family can be a forewarning of depression. Depression is not merely another aspect of the loss of sexual arousal. Depression can aggravate any medical condition and without doubt makes life seem negative and unpleasant. But did you know that depression could also affect your hormones?

David, a young man in South Carolina smoked constantly. He wrote in an email to me, "I have been experiencing symptoms such as fatigue, lack of motivation, severe depression, loss of sensation throughout my entire body, memory loss, difficulty concentrating, visual acuity and especially loss of male sexual features such as strong voice, body strength, motor function controls, warm comfortable sensations, feeling of sexual arousal, etc." David blamed his depression and low sex drive on his low testosterone.

David had suffered from depression for a year and a half. "I believe my testosterone levels are low," he continued, "I can't even get interested in my girlfriend." For David, a diagnosis of low testosterone levels would be a relief. "I'm hoping my levels are low because I know there is a treatment for this," he said. "It is hard to believe it could be a hormone problem since I am only 19, but anything is possible."

Is it really possible that David could have low testosterone levels at the tender age of 19? David's physical symptoms could be caused by other factors such as depression or an inadequate diet or some hereditary condition. Few young men at 19 experience testosterone deficiency unless they abuse alcohol, marijuana and nicotine, or all three during their formative years.

David doesn't seem to know what's causing his dejection. In his correspondence with me, he didn't see any connection between his gloominess and his habit of smoking two packs a day plus his heavy use of alcohol, (one to two six-packs of beer every day.) When he came to see me, David was slovenly dressed and his personal hygiene was non-existent. I suspected that David's depression was directly linked to nicotine and alcohol dependence. Dependence on drugs is a common sign of depression.

Depression is a serious condition. We all get up on the wrong side of the bed from time to time, but we snap out of it as the day goes on. Not so with people who are suffering from clinical depression.

For these people, sad feelings linger for weeks, months, even years. An incident such as a parking ticket or sharp words from the boss may trigger the shame, and depressed people are weighed down by a sense of doom and despair long after the occurrence has faded from memory.

What about David and Steve? Are they basically depressed? Steve is showing symptoms of "anhedonia," the medical term for the "absence of happiness" an identifying characteristic of depression. As a depressed person, Steve is a victim of the most common mood-related disorder in the world and his life is on hold unless he can get treated and overcome his problem. In much the same way, David suffers from drug dependence and loss of his sex drive, a serious situation for any adolescent.

Worldwide, depression is the fourth leading cause of disability and leading cause of adolescent death in the form of suicide, according to the World Health Organization (WHO) and is increasing at a rapid rate. In Western countries, one out of three people have endured at least one episode of depression and one out of five of people so affected have chronic, recurring depression. Approximately 11 to 15 percent kill themselves.

One study estimated the *annual* burden on the US economy at over $43 Billion, a depressing amount of money in an economy that depends on workers to focus on getting the job done. Disheartened workers are sick more often, see the doctor more often and enter hospitals more often. Depression alone costs more than all other chronic diseases *combined*, including heart disease, HIV/AIDS and other infections. These costs exceed a staggering *one third* of the US trillion dollar national health care budgets.

Older people are hit hardest by depression. One out of four Americans over the age of 65 suffers from the condition. Young Americans are not exempt. One out of 33 children and one out of eight adolescents puts up with clinical depression. The tragedy is that thousands of depressed children and teenagers are overlooked by our schools, and families are left to suffer on their own without adequate diagnosis or treatment. Youngsters are especially likely to fall through the cracks if they have a condition called bipolar depression, known as a "manic-depressive personality"; a disorder associated with rapid mood swings from elation to despair. Regrettably, the problem is routinely chalked up to "just another part of growing up."

Untreated depression can be deadly. At any age, depression brings about physical problems and drains people's sexual vitality and energy. Depressed people are more likely to experience substance abuse, financial losses, divorce and suicide. They can make others uncomfortable by seeming to complain about everything and they experience problems in every organ of their body. On the other hand, what physicians have learned recently is that the brains of victims of depression start to shrink and deteriorate the longer their depression goes untreated.

If your husband has a medical problem, depression can make it worse. Heart disease and other chronic conditions such as asthma, diabetes, arthritis and cancer are more than depressed people can bear. Depression may initiate these problems directly or merely leads to unhealthy behaviors, like smoking and drinking, with somber consequences.

Classic symptoms of clinical depression include sleeping too much or too little and trouble controlling one's appetite or one's finances. This is not the same as failing to balance your checkbook. Depressed individuals are still not paying bills when creditors are at their door. Ultimately, they develop serious work-related problems, frustrating friendships and failed sexual relationships. Most of the time, they live alone.

We use humor to brighten the darkness of despair. Many comedians admit to depressive episodes throughout their lives. Serious drama expands beyond humor to deal with the tragedies of suicide, addictions and despair. We'd much rather watch TV or read about it than deal with the reality of depression in our own lives. It feels much easier to ease the persistent worry by focusing on characters on the screen or the page. Escaping from reality is a common pastime for depressed folk.

Most depressed people do not understand that the cause of their depression is an imbalance in their brain chemistry. Instead, they assume they're depressed because they didn't deal effectively with stress in their lives. They feel the depression is their fault or the fault of somebody else that has mistreated them, for example. People with a strong religious orientation are more likely to feel guilty for surrendering to their depression. Occasionally doctors, who should know better, go along with the idea that self-discipline is the best way to cure depression, or maybe it's related to the patient's shortcoming.

Dr. Lundt declares, "All of us feel blue at times, but major depression results in profoundly dark moods frequently marked by uncontrolled crying, low energy levels, difficulty concentrating and poor motivation to get things done. Suicide is an ever-present risk." Depression is dreadfully intense and affects millions. But depression is a treatable medical condition.

Not realizing that there is a biological cause of depression, friends of depressed people often assume they can help with a little "pep talk" or positive reinforcement to boost self-esteem. Partners of depressed people often have the fantasy that if the other person would only stop complaining, everything would be all right. This shortsighted strategy never works. It only ends up raising the frustration level for anyone concerned, especially the patient.

To combat the lack of understanding about depression, pharmaceutical companies and mental health organizations sponsor mass media campaigns to educate the public. Their efforts are admirable because without proper information, too many parents, teachers and health care providers don't understand what their loved one might be fighting. They fail to recognize the symptoms of depression or assume that depression is easily overcome with the exercise of a little "will power" or a new interest.

One of my patients, Dianne, a 33-year-old homemaker, shared with me the reality of depression and its effect on her life." I have been unhappy and extremely irritable for a long time now," she told me. "I have no patience with friends and family. I have little or no interest in any of the things or people that used to interest me. I feel like crying entirely too often and I do cry over ridiculous things. My appetite has decreased. I'm having a difficult time getting a good night's sleep. I've tried to ignore these symptoms for too long. I feel embarrassed to admit that I have a problem, though there's no doubt in my mind that I do. I feel sorry for my family. They have to deal with my moodiness and inattentiveness. I can see that it is affecting their behavior as well. When I had a flat tire three days ago, I began crying and became terrified that I wouldn't be able to stop. Over a flat tire! That was the last straw, as they say. Please give me some advice. I need it."

For Dianne and persons like her, depression sucks the joy from life like a leech sucking blood. The depressed person, seeing no hope for change, may consider suicide as the only option that makes sense. If someone feels lost and hopeless, isn't taking an antidepressant enough? What does depression have to do with hormones?

Our adrenal glands release several hormones on a predictable daily basis. Can any of these cause depression? One of these hormones, *cortisol,* also known as "the stress hormone" is secreted whenever we feel anxious or distressed. This hormone helps our bodies cope with an emergency by increasing our ability to make glucose, the brain's primary source of fuel.

Throughout the day levels of cortisone increase and subside in a predictable rhythmic pattern of the "cortisol cycle." The normal cortisol cycle peaks at about 8 a.m. and again at about 4 p.m. When you woke up this morning, the act of waking up triggered a surge of cortisol that boosted you out of bed. A good number of people suffering from depression receive their first burst of cortisol about three o'clock in the morning. They wake up startled and often have trouble going back to sleep. No wonder they usually feel worse when it's time to get up. The day starts with increased anxiety and mood disturbances and then the cycle starts repeats when they have trouble falling asleep, only to awaken too early.

Evidence suggests that the corticotropin-releasing factor (CRF) from the pituitary gland regulates our cortisol levels so that we can cope with stress in our daily lives. But if the levels get too high, cortisol can become incredibly destructive. This unremitting stress, such as divorce or the death of a loved one, leads to an overactive response, throwing our entire system into turmoil.

People who are severely depressed not only tend to have a higher concentration of CRF in their spinal fluid but many of these people have more CRF-producing brain cells. Research studies link the production of additional CRF to chronic stress. This occurs only with ongoing stress that does not let up, such as torture, grief, or divorce. Consequently the CRF production goes into overcapacity. High CRF levels disturb the delicate balance of the adrenal system, controlled by the pituitary.

Today pharmaceutical companies are looking at CRF-blocking drugs that show promise in bringing relief to depressed persons. These drugs could be more effective than many of today's medicines, which are aimed at increasing the action of the "happy, energetic, pleasure promoting" neurotransmitters: dopamine and norepinephrine. These medications replaced many of the specific serotonin reuptake inhibitors that were considered the "calming, sleepy, nighttime" neurotransmitters. There are many as yet undiscovered subtypes of each of these groups of biological molecules.

The neurotransmitters are special chemicals in the brain that make it possible for nerve cells to "talk" to each other. Too few or too many cause depression or make it better. In some cases the language of the brain becomes twisted into a negative, shameful, scolding voice that makes the life worse. Negative talk and worry are far more common in depression.

How you deal with stress is related to the way your brain is "wired."

Each of us must have a balance of neurotransmitters to handle any stressful situation that is out of our control. These same neurotransmitters empathize with your hormone levels. When you become depressed, your neurotransmitters are not up to dealing with the simple stressors of life. With each episode of depression, the amount of stress needed to upset your life becomes less and less. Symptoms may come and go but the depression is unending.

Why Do Hormones Malfunction during Depression?

All humans are plagued by stress, but the hormone that gets most of the attention for being associated with stress is still cortisol, "the stress hormone." Basically, here's the explanation as to why cortisol makes people feel depressed.

During times of stress, cortisol from the adrenals converts proteins to glucose, the major source of energy for your brain. The resulting burst of glucose gives you energy to deal with the stressful situation. Divorce, death of a loved one, retirement or financial loss carries a heavier load of constant anxiety that can override the cortisol-regulating mechanism. Unvarying stress in the long run gives rise to elevated cortisol levels that lead to confusion, dizziness, memory loss and a weakened immune system. The higher CRF levels rise, the more likely dysfunction will result.

Cortisol responds to the day-night cycle we call the circadian rhythm. Levels of cortisol normally peak between 7 and 8 a.m. when we're getting out of bed to face the day. Bright light signals the sudden discharge of brain histamine, which activates cortisol, waking us up. Super high cortisol stifles both brain and tissue histamines. Therefore, as part of depression, the sleep-awake cycles are disrupted. At night, the hormone, melatonin, responds to darkness and reverses the wakening effect of cortisol.

Dehydroepiandrosterone, or DHEA, another major adrenal hormone, has a different developmental history. Its numbers increase rapidly during childhood, reaching a peak in youth and then decline thereafter. DHEA concentration is reduced in major depressive disorders for both adolescents and adults. DHEA, in contrast to cortisol, has brain-protective action, reducing the toxic effects of cortisol on our thinking. DHEA may thus have a beneficial role in the "alternative" treatment of depression. According to Dr. Owen Wolkowitz at Langley-Porter Psychiatric Institute, DHEA activity provides a perfect example of how two hormones with directly opposite effects can restore the balance in our brain.

This push-me-pull-you interaction of melatonin, DHEA, testosterone and cortisol is typical of how most hormones network against/ with each other. You may have an idea of what happens when hormones become imbalanced when you see a fight between a small dog and a bigger one. The larger animal can grab the small one by the throat and shake it to death. Overproduction of a single potent hormone can quash the action of a less potent, but no less important one. You might speculate what factors would cause such an inequality in the first place.

It may surprise you to realize that visible light can act like that big dog, shaking melatonin into submission. Bright computer screens or partying into the late night hours can hinder melatonin from reaching its usual nighttime high. This visual over-stimulation prohibits melatonin from disabling the *cortisol effect* so we can awaken clear-headed the next morning. A lifestyle with carousing or work extending into the early hours of the morning consequently starts a delayed release of melatonin leading to cortisol activation at night instead of during the day.

After a few days, the sleep-wake cycles automatically adjust. People who continue with nighttime work will develop a pattern of waking up in the middle of the night regardless of when they go to bed. The next day they will feel exhausted. For those schedules requiring sleep during the daytime, cortisol levels can be held steady by shutting out light with heavy blinds or by wearing blinders. This reinforcement of the melatonin response allows them to sleep during the day. Unfortunately, when they wake up at night after sleeping during daylight hours, they miss the cortisol boost that is triggered by morning light and again feel lousy, confused and disoriented. Night after night of tossing and turning can bring on mood disorders like depression. We are all tied to the light bathing our planet.

One of the other profound biochemical consequences of depression is a steady increase in cortisol and a decrease in DHEA. But too little cortisol is also harmful. Some up-to-the-minute studies show that cortisol levels are low in people who suffer from a condition known as post-traumatic stress disorder having been exposed to a frightening situation. In these cases, poor sleep, explosive anger and depression can result. Imagine an exhausted, angry man thrashing around in his bed constantly awakened by nightmares and flashbacks.

This build up of cortisol suppresses erections by decreasing testosterone levels. This demonstrates another example of the opposing hormone negatively affecting its exact opposite. The combination of loss of sexual interest and sleep problems occurs in women too, after something as inconsequential as a minor car accident. How can you tell if you have too much or too little cortisol?

Tests on saliva collected at different times of the day have proven to be a sensitive indicator of an abnormal cortisol/DHEA pattern. Measuring cortisol levels in morning saliva is helpful as a screening test for depression. If treated early, such cortisol deficiencies can be corrected with DHEA supplemental therapy to stop the depression from progressing.

Many patients with dangerously high cortisol levels may benefit from testosterone or estrogen supplementation. Medical research suggests that testosterone has positive effects on mood and that raising its levels to normal will suppress the production of excess cortisol, reducing the chance of depression. DHEA supplementation in women has been found to increase both estrogen and testosterone readings and has been used in treating depression after menopause.

In clinical surveys, patients diagnosed with depression and associated hormonal imbalances who were treated with testosterone (T) reported that they not only felt better but also had more energy, better sexual function and improved moods. Could testosterone therapy offer a new treatment for depression?

Two research papers using testosterone to treat depression showed conflicting results. In a Columbia University six-week study, the researcher found little difference between the depression of low T patients who were given weekly T injections or placebo injections. He did notice however that his sexual function improved with testosterone.

Another eight-week study at McLean Hospital included men with low or borderline testosterone. A significant improvement in unresponsive depression was observed and linked to an increase in the levels of circulating *free* testosterone. The patient applied a transdermal testosterone gel that will be discussed in more detail later in this book.

These studies confirm that low levels of testosterone can lead to negative moods and reduce mental acuity. Depression does not discriminate against age or profession. Losing that sharpness and quick response is universally seen in aging persons as their hormone levels dwindle, but this is not the same as depression. A physician trained in detecting this all-encompassing condition must first make the diagnosis.

As I mentioned earlier, the reason women seem to suffer from depression more than men may be that they talk about their feelings. This is good for them because the earlier depression is recognized, the sooner it can be diagnosed and treated. Alternatively, men apparently want to bolster their invincibility or don't like to complain to their doctors about anything as personal as their emotions. When they feel depressed, men often turn to self-medicating with alcohol or street drugs only to slide into a deeper depression. The condition could quickly become impossible for a spouse to handle by herself.

In desperation, men too often take their own lives when they can no longer deal with the overwhelming feelings of despair. Four times as many men as women commit suicide, according to data analyzed by the American Association of Suicidology, an organization dedicated to preventing suicide in the United States. This association also comments that each year nearly 30,000 people decide to commit suicide in the US and succeed in their attempt. For every suicide there are from 8 to 25 attempts that do not result in death.

Why would anyone welcome death? Locked in depression, people feel as if their life is slipping away and that they have nothing to look forward to but the inevitability of death. It's a dismal picture. They think it will end their suffering. But this position may be totally reversed with antidepressants.

This point is equally important for women and the men who love them. Keep in mind that depression is predominantly a disease of mental imbalance linked to a shortage of the specific chemicals known as neurotransmitters. In this book, I will only discuss five of these chemical messengers: serotonin, dopamine, norepinephrine, adrenaline and nitric oxide.

How Do Antidepressants Work?

Several neurotransmitters are involved in depression and most of the older medications only affected one type. Antidepressant medications have existed for over 30 years, but they don't work for everyone. Older medications affected only a single neurotransmitter family. Newer medicines are capable of increasing the levels of serotonin, dopamine *and* norepinephrine. These dual-acting meds cause fewer side effects and produce a better therapeutic effect than older variety.

They aren't cheap. The newer antidepressants are the single largest item in the total US pharmacy budget. But the costs of not treating depression are much greater! Sorry to say, it sometimes comes down to a choice between poverty and sanity.

Depression also co-exists with other health problems. For example, a patient who is hospitalized for any reason ranging from heart disease to cancer has an incidence of depression ranging from 20 to 42 percent. This is important information to share with your spouse. Most patients with diseases of the nervous system are depressed, for example the incidence of depression in the various diseases ranges from:

Heart Attacks and Stroke	35.0%
Epilepsy	55.0%
Parkinson's	51.0%
Cushing's (or abnormally high cortisol levels)	83.0%
Multiple sclerosis	55.0%
Alzheimer's	11.0%

Most depressed people have no clue that a chemical imbalance could be the cause of their unhappiness. They find the cause for their sadness in the problems of their lives such as feeling uncontrollable grief or breaking up with a girlfriend or a boyfriend. Crying all the time to mourn the death of someone dear to you or not wanting to get out of bed because you hate school or your job could all be signs of a depressive illness. It's not uncommon for depressed persons to feel "crazy" or "out of control," when the root of the problem is a neurotransmitter imbalance. Depression is far more severe and intense than a bad mood. Today the "nervous breakdown" some folks used to dread can be treated with appropriate medications before it takes place.

Diagnosis is the most important aspect of this disorder since it cannot be treated until it has been diagnosed. General practitioners need to stop rushing through clinical consultations with their patients and take the time to spot early signs of depression. The doctor's index of suspicion should materialize whenever patients repeatedly complain of not feeling right or experiencing rapid mood swings.

If a person responds quickly to a new antidepressant drug, but the medicine loses its potency in a relatively short time, it may be that this person has the bipolar type of depression. Another symptom presents as the patient who returns to a doctor's office more than a dozen times a year but is not on any long-term treatment program requiring such frequent visits. A person with a close relative (parent, grandparent, or sibling) who has a mood disorder is more likely to become a victim of the same thing. But even patients without family members diagnosed with clinical depression, can start to experience negative feelings in late childhood or adolescence. The interruption of regular sleep patterns can present a clue.

Hormones become valuable in counteracting the disruption of the circadian rhythms that occur with depression. Depression and sexual dysfunction relate to each other in a time-dependent fashion. In other words, one leads the other follows. Additionally, the intensity of the depression can vary depending on the time of day, week, or month. Like a roller coaster ride, depression is not always downhill.

Stress may be unavoidable in today's world. But if you or someone you love has depressed relatives, prolonged trauma or untreated depression can lead to dementia; life is tough. Regaining control in your life can help you cope with stress, but sometimes medication and counseling are necessary.

Nervous tension takes its toll on the regulating system in the brain. The memory terminal of the hippocampus, located between the hypothalamus and the pituitary gland, begins to malfunction after only a few months of constant worry. As over 90 percent of the serotonin receptors are in the hippocampus, stress can lead to memory loss with a shrinking hippocampus. People with dementia have shrunken brains on autopsy. So it pays to be proactive and get your depression treated before it's too late.

The irony of depression is that those who suffer the most from its effects may be the least aware of its presence in their lives. If the disease has caused the person, usually a man, to lose his ability to experience pleasure, he may also lack the insight to realize that he has a problem. You can't help a person who thinks nothing is wrong. It is for this reason that wives and friends of depressed men get so frustrated. They know something is terribly wrong but the men won't admit it or refuse treatment. Don't let this stop you from trying.

Mid-life Crisis and Male Andropause

Whenever I speak to women about the men in their lives, they want to know why men don't ask for help. They tell me that when their boyfriends or husbands are having trouble with heart problems, depression, impotence or a myriad of other problems, they hate to complain, much less visit a doctor. Women want to know how they can help their men make positive changes. The best time to get involved is when your man is going through male menopause, a condition now referred to as Viropause and Andropause or in Canada they call it Partial Androgen Deficiency in Aging Men (PADAM).

I tell these women that andropause is the medical name of a male syndrome consisting of the consequences of aging plus other physical, sexual and psychological symptoms. Men going through andropause suffer from weakness, fatigue, and reduced muscle or bone mass. Other symptoms include: sexual dysfunction, depression, anxiety, irritability plus insomnia with associated impairment of memory.

Of course women get changes in their hormone levels as well. The difference is that the transition for a woman is shorter and prompts her to seek help much more aggressively than a man. Menopause, announced by the end of menstrual periods, takes place in most women 45 to 55 years of age. In men, the process of hormone depletion is long and complicated by testosterone fluctuations over many decades. In other words, andropause is a prolonged process leading to decades of suffering. The Massachusetts Aging Study in 2005 described a drop in men's testosterone from ages 40 to 69.

Only recently have researchers begun to focus on the "male menopause." This term loosely applies to the mid-life crisis that men reach in their late fifties or early sixties. Some doctors do not believe andropause, though the word first appeared in the medical literature as far back as 1952, when it was defined as "the natural cessation of the sexual function in older men." Notice two points in this definition:

(1) Andropause was considered "natural."
(2) It was assumed that sexual function should cease at a certain point in a man's life.

Neither of these assumptions is true.

Men and women adjust to increasing depression and sexual dysfunction associated with advancing years in vastly different ways. Women, for example, go through "the change" rather abruptly, while for aging men the decline in hormones is slower and hardly noticeable over time. The slow course and unpredictability of andropause contribute to its lack of recognition and its dismissal as nothing but a sign of "normal" aging.

Think about that the next time you hear an acquaintance being described as a "grumpy old man." Consider the possibility that he is not grumpy at all but simply entering andropause. Hormones may play a significant role in the mid-life crisis of all men. Let's take a closer look at how this works.

As time goes by, hormone deficiencies generally cause failing memories, more irritability and fatigue, symptoms similar to depression. The physical signs of aging include the progression of blood vessel diseases, varicose veins, thinning of the skin and hair, high blood pressure and increasing cholesterol levels.

There's more! Some of the obvious signs of andropause include: progressive aging of the face, development of a potbelly, loss of pubic hair, shrinking of sexual organs, balding, increasing ear and nose hair and loss of muscle or skin tone. These occur in the majority of men as they age. Are hormones involved?

Over the years several hormones, especially testosterone, become depleted, leading to a deficiency. The good news is that just as women with menopausal symptoms respond well to hormone replacement therapy, males experiencing andropause can also be treated effectively with hormones.

When it comes to sexual function, the natural aging process is not "natural" at all. As men pass through their fifties and sixties, their andropause is commonly associated with a decrease in sexual motivation. This leads to lack of interest in sex compounded by both ejaculatory and urinary problems. Many men suffering with low testosterone should not accept this as part of normal aging. Neither should women allow this in their mates.

These men are only manifesting early warning signs of a more serious problem. Testosterone deficiency diseases are showing up in men as young as 30 to 40 and in women of the same age group. What happens to men when they lose their ability to get an erection? Alarming statistics from recent research suggest that men who become impotent—unable to develop an erection—die about 20 years earlier than other men, usually from some type of heart disease.

As a matter of fact, the heart is a huge target organ for hormone imbalances. A study in 1988 by the well-known hormone researcher Conrad Swartz confirmed the fact that total testosterone levels are much lower in men with severe heart disease than in healthy men. Total serum testosterone levels were found to be *100 points lower* in patients who had suffered a heart attack than in those who had not. Once a man becomes totally impotent (no erections), he loses his zeal for life. Subsequently or simultaneously, he loses his libido, his muscle mass, his mental acuity fades and depression sets in.

By 80 years, three out of four men are impotent. At 40 years of age, roughly one third of the male population is unable to achieve an erection at will. The only encouraging detail here is that one out of four men in his eighties or older is *not* impotent. Many men live out their lives to an old age without ever losing their sexual prowess. If andropause were "natural" wouldn't every man experience its effects?

While andropause is not synonymous with impotence, it is usually associated with loss of libido and sexual function. Problems related to andropause may be caused by a deficiency of multiple hormones including growth hormone, DHEA, thyroxine, melatonin and oxytocin and the primary male androgens, testosterone, androstenedione and DHT. The good news is that men can retain potency and enjoy good sex as often as twice a week, well into their nineties, despite age-related drop in hormone levels.

You may wonder, "What is the secret to sexual longevity?" Male sexuality does not just end at a certain age. We need to pay attention to two facts about male sexuality:

(1) More and more men are living into their nineties or beyond.
(2) In developed countries fertility rates for men of all ages are declining.

What is happening to your boyfriend or husband? Are they testosterone deprived?

A program of testosterone supplementation portioned out in individually adjusted doses will increase sexual drive and improve function in any man. Testosterone replacement therapy will provide more lean body mass, improve insulin sensitivity, enhance anti-clotting action and expand blood vessels to reduce blood pressure. These sound like important reactions and good reasons to consider getting your mate tested.

Even so, despite enormous medical progress over the past few decades, the final years of life are still accompanied by increasing ill health, depression and disability. This does not have to happen to you if you are able to find a doctor to help you and your loved ones keep your hormones balanced. Hormone replacement for men may one day be as common as hormone replacement for women. Many of the problems men experience during their so-called mid-life crises, such as diminished energy and vitality, irritability, trouble concentrating and decreased muscle strength, could simply be the result of declining hormones and not "old age."

Sexual Dysfunction and Depression

Sexual dysfunction refers to a lack of sexual desire or difficulty in achieving arousal, climax, or ejaculation. This condition affects about 75 million Americans and the numbers are rising! One common cause of sexual dysfunction is depression. Depressed people tend to avoid sex! Either they cannot perform the sex act in a normal manner or they lack the passion. Anxiety about a man's sexual performance can actually produce sexual dysfunction, even if, in most cases, there is a physical difficulty related to blood flow.

Failure to achieve erections and the lack of interest in someone who has been a sexual partner are indications of depression. Loss of early morning erections should be taken as an early warning sign of a hormone shorage. Wives and girlfriends should be quite concerned because men with these problems are at risk for much more serious outcome than simply the lack of erections.

If you or someone you know is depressed, you may be familiar with the symptoms as they affect your own sexlife. Yet, if you have never been severely depressed, the facts about any mood disorders may elicit a yawn or a shrug. So some people are depressed. No surprises there. Sure some men have trouble getting it up. What else is new? We all know some women can be sexually frigid. Maybe they just don't love their husbands. Maybe he's a jerk. Maybe she's being too critical.

The truth is that depression is a disease of denial and the reality is that too many people are suffering from this condition without knowing what's wrong. Though sexual dysfunction is a dependable indicator of impending depression, these hints are easily ignored by busy doctors and by deteriorating patients.

Excuses abound but if someone has no interest, they try not to think about sex. Patients with depression are simply told that they need to see a marriage counselor or take a vacation. By the time depression advances to the final stages, regarding a loss of any interest in love or even in life, it's too late. Suicide is a real threat.

When patients describe the sudden onset of volatile moods over which they have no control, a red flag should go up. These patients are trying to give us a clue to their problem. Physicians must be sensitive to their patient's body language and vocabulary.

The loss of libido is a common indicator of clinical depression. Does depression cause sexual dysfunction or is it the other way around? A good way to answer this question is to listen to a patient's story. I remember talking to Michael, a math teacher in Chicago, regarding his frustration with a medical visit.

Michael watched his testosterone drop over a few months from 550 to 270 ng/dl, as his energy and sexual feelings shut down. He was dissatisfied when both his urologist and personal physician put him off, by reassuring him that his condition was either his unfortunate lot in life or just part of the aging process.

A young 41-year-old, Michael was physically active, playing full court basketball and running without much fatigue for long periods of time. His only health problem was high blood pressure, for which he was taking 20 milligrams of Lotrel, an antihypertensive, to hold it in check. His identical twin brother had a similar problem with high blood pressure.

Michael's testosterone score was well below the normal range and he was still fairly young. Did he get treated? No. His doctor didn't ask about his family history, though the fact that Michael's twin brother had high blood pressure suggested a hereditary basis for his problem. His doctor was aware that hypertension is a valid predictor of early heart disease. Michael's high blood pressure should have been investigated further before he was handed a prescription for a bottle of blood pressure pills.

The more medications the doctor adds to his treatment plan without a correct diagnosis, the greater the likelihood Michael's sexual problems will increase. Sometimes medical doctors continue to add more blood pressure medications when a single agent isn't adequate, overlooking testosterone deficiency or a genetic factor as the cause of the sexual problem.

As a rule, a doctor's next step would have been to consider the possibility that Michael has a hidden testosterone deficiency. What should Michael do if he continues to suffer with no help from his urologist or his general internist? Should he see another doctor? What if he can't find anyone on his health plan that believes low testosterone may be playing a role in his hypertension or his sexual difficulty?

This scenario is not that far-fetched. Michael will probably give up in frustration and like many men take matters into his own hands. He may consult the Internet, ordering a testosterone preparation available without a doctor's prescription. Not only could Michael end up with a totally ineffective, counterfeit testosterone product, or worse, a dangerous oral anabolic steroid.

Unsupervised prescription sales over the Internet are all too prevalent and lay the groundwork for a tragedy waiting to happen. I believe in free speech and support the marvelous power of the Web, but I believe that this feature of the World Wide Web needs regulating. Just because you read something on the Internet does not mean it's true. There is no substitute for a qualified physician in treating hormone inadequacy. I urge you to reject the numerous tidbits of misinformation that are often circulated on the web. If you have any trouble finding a good doctor, check with a good medical school or university in your region.

In spite of adequate exercise, Mike reported a drop in his testosterone level and a discouragingly low sex drive. Testosterone therapy would probably help Michael lower his blood pressure and feel like a man again. Too many doctors treat symptoms instead of searching for the root cause of the disorder. The reasoning that a thorough investigation would take too much time or cost too much money is absurd. Don't let your husband fall for that line.

Without a correct diagnosis and an understanding doctor, men in Michael's shoes give up on doctors and opt for the dangerous route of self-medication. They don't recognize that they may be the victims of an incomplete diagnosis. Trying to solve the problem with more and more medication and treating only the signs and symptoms does not address the underlying cause.

Another anecdote involves, Gina, a 51-year-old Italian female, married for 20 years who was ready to call it quits. "My Antonio has no interest in sex. I do all I can to look attractive, I even took up golf and still he doesn't want to get close. We used to have such a good sex life and now, nothing! Maybe there is something wrong with me? " Gina's estrogen and progesterone levels were totally normal and she had seen her gynecologist a few months earlier. Yet when I tested Gina's testosterone levels they were far below normal, so I started her on a bioidentical testosterone supplement. After 30 days, she returned to report no changes except for a happy note that she had lost a few pounds without dieting.

I explained that it usually takes some time for testosterone to become effective as a sexual stimulant. A month later she came back with a huge smile on her face. "It's working," she said, "like being on our honeymoon again." A correct diagnosis makes all the difference!

Premature Ejaculation—the Unspoken Fear.

Many men avoid sex because they are concerned they will lose their erection or climax before their partner has been satisfied. This fear is one of man's most common sexual concerns—"premature ejaculation" or ejaculating earlier than desired. About 25 percent of men experience repeated poor control over ejaculation. This condition affects men at any point in their lives. Of course, any apprehension or panic during intercourse will interrupt the process, as you would expect resulting in loss of an erection.

"Premature ejaculation is defined as persistent or recurrent ejaculation with minimal sexual stimulation before, upon, or shortly after penetration, or before the person wishes, causing distress and embarrassment to one or both partners, potentially affecting sexual relationships and overall

well-being." (Ortho-McNeil Pharmaceutical Inc. statement made on 10/26/2004)

ALZA Corporation is developing a new drug, *dapoxetine*, for treating premature ejaculation. Dapoxetine is actually a short-acting serotonin reuptake inhibitor. It is interesting to note that all anti-depressants in the SRI-family, delay ejaculation when they are used for treating depression. For this reason new antidepressants that act on multiple neurotransmitters have been developed to put a stop to sexual dysfunction. Some of these newer agents—NRIs or nor-epinephrine reuptake inhibitors such as Wellbutrin XL® seem to in-crease sexual drive in women. Others affect the entire range of neu-rotransmitters and may be more effective without sexual side effects.

The Secret to Treating Depression Successfully

Depressed people tend to take one of two positions: they either be-lieve they have a physical problem and the doctor does not know what it is, or are convinced that they are fine and that those around them are sick. This is denial at its deepest level. The first step in treating any type of depression is for the individual suffering from its effects to accept they have a problem. If a person believes instead that some life circumstance is dictating his or her moods, it will be next to impossible to change that person's mind and get them to take their medication.

Once the doctor and patient focus on the depression and elimi-nate other important issues as the root cause of the person's problem, they can work together to achieve total relief from the disease. Recov-ery and the correction of hormone imbalance should be the goal.

You may recall that in depression the hypothalamus, deep within the brain, stops functioning normally. The hypothalamus influences our memories and emotions and regulates our adrenals and many other hormone glands. When hyperactivity of the adrenal system elevates levels of cortisol, the stress hormone, this brings on symptoms of depression accompanied by aches and pains in addition to unpleasant moods. High cortisol levels overpower our nervous system, especially the hypothalamus and the entire human organism becomes unbalanced. This mechanism is the current explanation for why people get depressed.

Dr. Leslie Lundt evaluates some of the new medications developed for mood disorders and talks about the search for the "perfect pill." She writes, "If we don't live in a perfect world, it's not because the drug companies aren't trying. A whole new class of medications has been developed to deal with troublesome moods and other mental problems. They're called psychotropic medications and their use is climbing rapidly. Antidepressants, one category of psychotropic medications, are now a 20 billion dollar industry in the US. A 1997 study showed that nearly eight out of ten persons being treated for depression received some kind of psychotropic medication as part of their treatment."

I have already discussed why women are particularly prone to sad moods, bipolar disorder or low levels of depression. Depression is not a simple disease but the first step in treating this complex disorder is to sort out the type of depression we are dealing with so that the doctor can implement a successful treatment plan. There are many antidepressants and many different levels of depression.

A doctor who recognizes the role that hormones play in depression might prescribe a combination of an antidepressant plus a thyroid hormone, for example, to correct an unresponsive depression. In some women estrogen plus an antidepressant is more effective than either agent alone. The improvement in many men's depressive symptoms after adding supplemental hormone therapy with testosterone supports this approach for many patients.

There are many methods of treating depression medically. Alan Michaels, a California medical researcher, discovered that elderly people with depression are sometimes deficient in the hormone DHEA. But low levels of practically any hormone will induce some depression in either sex. Owen Wolkowitz, a psychiatrist at the University of California at San Francisco, has successfully treated depression in people who did not respond to other therapies, with high doses of pharmaceutical-grade DHEA. Dr. Lund uses Provigil, a histamine activator, in combination with antidepressants to induce rapid remission of depression. My psychotherapist friend uses cognitive therapy and no medication. Obviously there are many techniques available for the treatment of this disease.

While DHEA or testosterone works for some depressed patients, nearly nine out of ten people respond well to one of the newer dual-action antidepressant medications like Effexor® or venlafaxine. Dual-acting agents, such as duloxetine or Cymbalta®, are often superior to either serotonin or norepinephrine inhibitors. These new combination drugs have fewer side effects and seem to help more people than the older agents. According to psychiatrists, the levels must be adjusted up slowly to suit each individual. Occasionally, none of the antidepressants work because of differences between people and the various types of depression. In these cases a combination of medications, including lithium or other mood stabilizers, may be helpful.

You may wonder how doctors can find the *right* antidepressant. Sometimes patients feel as if it's simply a "trial-and-error" process. Thought we do not treat a major mental disorder by guesswork, a certain amount of trial-and-error is necessary. The goal in all types of depression therapy is *remission* or *total relief* from all symptoms. Remission of depression means a return to normal functioning, not simply a positive response to taking certain drugs. Treatment without remission of symptoms will surely lead to relapse and recurrences. While it is an elusive goal, remission is the gold standard of care in treating depression.

As the physical symptoms of depression: sleeplessness, lack of sexual arousal and abnormal cortisol levels diminish, a person's mental capabilities return. Those who do not achieve remission are three times as likely to suffer a relapse, three times as likely to become depressed again and just as likely to attempt suicide. Those who become involved in substance abuse are even more likely to experience a worsening of their depression than those who received non-addictive antidepressants.

The good news is that depression is one of the most treatable illnesses in medicine. Nearly all patients with depression begin to feel better after taking their medications. It has been said that all antidepressants are equally effective in terms of overall rate of response. But certain SRIs such as Paxil and Zoloft are short-acting and when stopped abruptly cause symptoms such as anxiety, headache, dizziness and severe depression. This condition is termed "discontinuation syndrome."

Other SRIs, like Prozac, stay in the system for weeks after stopping the meds. Most SRIs are not indicated in older women since they cause too many side effects. Some NRIs decrease appetite and increase sexual drive. Whatever the case, there is a medication that will work if the physician and patients are persistent in reaching for the goal of remission of the depression.

If the doctor's prescription doesn't work, patients sometimes turn to over-the-counter (OTC) remedies. Self-styled "natural antidepressant therapies" such as St. John's Wort, MSM and SAM-E are popular. Because they can buy these without a doctor's order, some people take all three! Many people seek out these supplements because they believe they can lift their depression and make them feel better. They may be "natural" from an herbal perspective, but they contain compounds that can act like drugs in the human system.

St. John's Wort or hypericum is prescribed as a serotonin stimulant in Germany. It relieves depression in some people, but in combination with SRIs it can create too much serotonin, a condition termed the "serotonin syndrome." A potentially lethal overdose of serotonin (5-HT) is associated with vomiting, loss of orientation and possibly death.

Even now over-the-counter hormones like melatonin and DHEA that anyone can buy without a prescription may help ease depression, but because of their close relationship to the functioning of other hormones circulating in our bodies, we should not play games using these drugs. Just because you can buy them at the drug store doesn't mean they're good for you or that they will work the way the advertisers claim.

If you really want to help your husband or significant other, advise them not to try to treat their own depression. Depression is a complicated disorder involving your brain, your chemical make-up, your hormonal system and your sense of who you are. The disease has so many facets that a physician must diagnose it correctly before any treatment is given. After the diagnosis is made, hormones and neurotransmitter levels must first be restored to a balanced state. Finally, a brief period of intense psychotherapy is essential to train the once depressed person to recognize triggers and personality quirks that encourage depression-associated thinking and behavior.

We know that hormonal and brain systems work differently in men and women in response to the same emotional experience. Obviously, it is quite important to consider the unique and changing biology of males and females when planning treatment for depression or a stress-related illness.

Thanks to miraculous advances in pharmacology, that branch of medicine that deals with the treatment of disease by using medications, a new life is available to those suffering from depression. Of course, the right prescription does no good unless the patient stays on the medicine program. There's a big temptation to stop taking pills especially after they begin working and the person starts to feel better.

Paying attention to your hormones is more important than knowing all the facts about mental diseases. A prevention-oriented check up plus a hormone screening can make the difference between health and future predicaments. Hormone balancing provides an important tool for physicians. If hormonal imbalance is your problem, new and convenient hormone delivery systems are available to help you obtain relief.

Testosterone Gels

Studies show that hormones can be absorbed through the skin and that levels of free testosterone increase with the use of testosterone gels. These gels are a quick and easy way for men to receive testosterone (T) replacement. Some men, do not do well with alcohol-based gels, possibly because of the low potency of the testosterone. Most of these gels contain only one percent testosterone, which means that at a ten percent absorption rate, the five-gram packets deliver about five milligrams of testosterone per day (the same as the testosterone output of a man's testicles).

"I have been on AndroGel for about a year and a half now due to hypogonadism," Richard wrote me from Chicago. "Before Andro-Gel, my T level was 210. After starting AndroGel at 5 milligrams per day, my level went up to 755. Six months ago it was down to 505 and my most recent test just last week it had dropped to 415. I'm starting to feel some of the old symptoms of low T: foggy thinking, low energy and low sex drive. Has anyone else had this problem with AndroGel becoming less effective? My doc says my T levels are still within the normal range. What can I do? "

Richard's dilemma may be due to inadequate hormone replacement. Some men require up to 10 grams of AndroGel per day for complete testosterone replacement therapy. The doctor should be careful about monitoring results and adjusting the dose of hormones. Correcting low hormone levels can put off suffering from decreased libido, or erectile dysfunction, but it isn't always possible to restore the balance of hormones with a standard dose of hormone supplement. Other hormones such as progesterone or DHEA might be required.

Men who receive restorative T therapy often describe feelings of heightened motivation, excitement, inspiration and a restoration of their passion for work and sex. Other benefits include a sense of confidence, freedom from fatigue and powerful, aggressive, but positive moods.

These are wonderful effects but please don't get me wrong, I don't want you to rush out and start using hormones thinking you can feel this way immediately. Different people respond differently to hormone replacement therapy because we each have unique hormonal or biochemical requirements.

In my practice, more patients arrive with depression or hormone imbalances than vitamin deficiencies. As a matter of fact, testosterone deficiency has become so common that it's no longer the exception but rather the rule. From my experience in over 30 years of clinical practice, I recommend that any man over 40 should have his hormone levels tested. Women can usually wait a decade later or after menopause to be checked.

Let's listen to Joe, a California construction worker, who sent me this classic description of the devastating consequences of testosterone deficiency: "I was just reading some testimonials on your website and it seemed like I was reading about myself. I'm tired of getting responses that I'm normal when I know there has been a huge change in my life. I feel like my virility has gone downhill. My sex life has been terrible. I have weak erections and lose them quickly. I have had these symptoms for at least a year now. I know it's not diabetes because I've been tested for that three times along with my testosterone levels, measured between 320 and 340," (normal range is 300-1200).

Joe was beginning to feel desperate. "My weight has ballooned from 175 to 245 pounds in a year and a half," he continued. "I know it's not a mental thing because I had the physical symptoms first and then gained weight. I don't feel like a 29-year-old man but more like one in his eighties who can't get it up and whose virility has disappeared. This has depressed me so much that I don't go anywhere and have no energy or motivation to work out like I used to. I'm too tired to exercise. I hope you can help me. I would be happy to drive to your office from Orange County."

Why does Joe feel like an old man? Joe is not yet 30 years old, yet he is complaining of a terrible sex life, weak erections, and a loss of his virility. Joe's testosterone level sits in the low normal range for his age. According to most medical providers, he should be fine, though he is obese. Many doctors would tell him the problem is not low testosterone, but rather a weight problem or too much stress. Are these doctors correct?

If Joe were in his sixties or seventies, nobody would be surprised by his low testosterone levels, which, on average, drop about 100 points for each decade of life. A young man like Joe should not have sexual dysfunction if he has a normal T level. Nevertheless, Joe knows his performance is far from normal. Something is not right. In Joe's case and he has plenty of company, total testosterone levels do not generally provide a useful measure of a man's sexual capacity. Joe's doctor needs to consider the more active forms of bioavailable and free testosterone as a *more accurate gauge* of hormonal function.

Doctors who measure only their patients' total testosterone levels are using the accepted standards but miss the diagnosis in men who could benefit from treatment. Reports from the Massachusetts Male Aging Study found that free testosterone was a *more sensitive* measure than total testosterone. The study revealed that while free testosterone drops by 1.4 percent per year and SHBG increases by 1.2 percent, total testosterone does *not* show a marked decrease with age.

Dr. Guay, one of the study's authors, points out that total testosterone decreases by about *0.4 percent each year,* so this does not reflect the true state of testosterone function. When free testosterone, which is normally 11 to 35 picograms per milliliter, drops below 7.4 picograms per milliliter, response to Viagra disappears. (A picogram is one trillionth of a gram.) Obviously, these infinitesimal amounts can have enormous consequences.

After numerous requests, Joe persuaded his doctor to check his free testosterone reading. "He pronounced me normal," he said, "but I still had all the signs of low testosterone levels: depression, lack of concentration, low libido and enlarged breasts. Finally, I demanded to see an endocrinologist who gave me a correct diagnosis of hypogonadism (deficient testosterone levels). He gave me an injection of testosterone and I began to feel better immediately. My smile returned and so did my sexual desire. I was so happy I had been persistent about my Catch-22."

But, all was not well. After overcoming this stumbling block, Joe's endocrinologist subsequently substituted a five-gram tube of Testim daily to which Joe did not respond as well. "I have been 'drunk' ever since," he told me. "I've had lots of side effects, but the main one is that I feel dazed and depressed most of the time. My eyes stay red and my friends think I'm impaired."

When he reported these side effects, the doctor tested his blood levels and found that his testosterone levels were higher than before but still in the low normal range. So he recommended 10 grams of the Testim gel each day. "I did so and am as drunk and confused as before but my eyes are redder than ever," Joe said. At this point Joe was not happy with Testim. He wanted to know what else he could do.

Joe's problem is not unique. Some men simply cannot tolerate the smell and flaky skin resulting from treatment with low potency T-gels. Regrettably, the alcohol base is necessary to dissolve the testosterone for transdermal delivery. Clinical trials at UCLA indicate that significantly larger volumes of AndroGel are needed to reach adequate testosterone concentrations for younger men. Though the gel can be applied to one site or several, large body areas must still be coated for adequate absorption.

Other factors must be playing a role in the effectiveness of testosterone in some men. Joe's testosterone readings seem fine, yet even now he complains of depression. Could a neurotransmitter deficiency be playing a confounding role in this mess?

Dopamine: Hormonal Rescue from Depression and Attention Deficit Disorder

A neurotransmitter named dopamine is essential for experiencing pleasure and arousal. A person who does not have enough dopamine experiences chronic fatigue, loss of libido and an overactive appetite. In addition, a lack of dopamine interferes with a person's ability to concentrate. Low dopamine levels are common in *anhedonia* and addictive behavior, in addition to depression or attention deficit disorder (ADD). Adults with ADD often consume huge quantities of caffeine or nicotine to stimulate dopamine.

But too much dopamine triggers weight loss, hallucinations, aggressive behavior and increased libido. In schizophrenics, mental patients who are not in touch with reality, dopamine saturates their brain. The excess dopamine creates actual images or voices termed *hallucinations* that do not really exist except in their minds.

According to Dr.Lundt, dopamine has positive benefits, "Dopamine increases a person's ability to concentrate and helps him or her feel motivated to stick to a task. Far more important in our drug-abusing culture, is the role of dopamine as the "reward element." A surge of dopamine in the brain brings about a feeling of accomplishment. The energy and sense of reward from the release of dopamine can be triggered by cocaine, encouraging the user to coke up again and again. The return is so intense that you can become addicted to cocaine after just one use. Other drugs of abuse, including amphetamines, also give the user a "high" by stimulating the release of dopamine."

Out of desperation, men with erectile or orgasmic problems sometimes turn to alcohol or street drugs to medicate their problem. Dopamine is stimulated by nicotine; one reason that depressed people and those who need extra ability to focus tend to be heavy cigarette smokers. The momentary pleasure they derive from nicotine in the cigarette is short lived and cravings for another puff soon follow.

Caffeine, speed, cocaine and methamphetamine are all powerful, habit-forming dopamine stimulants. By revving up the brain's dopamine production they banish any lingering wisps of anhedonia, producing invincible thoughts without the need for food or sleep. Of course, after days of sleep deprivation, other hormones fail and the addict "crashes."

Although dopamine aids concentration and suppresses appetite, it can lead to insomnia. Anyone who has tried a few cups of strong coffee at night knows this pretty well. The problem is that once the mind has been stimulated for hours or days, dopamine stores diminish and feelings of depression and worthlessness take over. This cycle drives a "speed addict" to repeatedly abuse this drug. The stress builds up, cortisol levels climb and before long the addict can no longer get high using the drug. Depression has taken over!

Problems can also take place when a person doesn't have enough dopamine in his or her body. Dopamine deficiency accounts for a number of psychiatric disorders.

"I have been caring for a son who has been diagnosed with bipolar depression with schizophrenic tendencies," Lisa wrote to me from Canada.

Besides being her son's sole support system, Lisa had to cope with legal issues that dragged on throughout an entire year. "His illness is so up and down and unpredictable," she said in her letter. "He has a therapist and a psychiatrist, but I have been the one everybody depends on to aid him. I will do it until the day I die."

Now Lisa is wondering about herself. "Lately, I cannot function like I usually do. I normally keep a spotless house, have dinner on the table, and am busy with lots of activities and friends. Now I look for any excuse NOT to be with my friends, I leave laundry in the dryer for days, I don't clean, I don't eat right, I can't sleep and I'm extremely edgy and moody."

Lisa thinks she may be depressed. "I have learned a lot about mental illness. I never felt it could hit me. I was the strongest. I was always up, the life of the party. Not any more. I can't tell you the last time I really enjoyed myself. I'm worried because I can't do anything about it. I can try to make a list of things to do around the house and even though I know they need to be done and though it is my nature to do these things without prompting, I just don't do any of them. I don't know how to explain that. I don't see sunshine anymore. I used to love the sun, but now I can't seem to find it even when it's shining above me."

Lisa has many problems in addition to depression. She feels she is not getting enough sunshine, which may be a metaphor for her lack of happiness. Lisa is probably suffering from "situational depression" or "burnout," which many caregivers experience when dealing with loved ones who are seriously ill.

Patients tormented by excessive fears and debilitating depression affect not only themselves but also their caregiver or spouse. Depression is not contagious, but caregivers often become depressed when they are involved with a loved one who is depressed or mentally ill and they may go on to develop full-blown clinical depression themselves.

Burnout taxes the victim emotionally and physically until the person simply shuts down. Caregivers with this problem may stop eating, stop sleeping and develop that flat emotional state, anhedonia. This type of depression is also common in children dealing with aging parents, frequently leading to chain smoking or drug abuse. Lisa's problem was probably caused by a deficiency in dopamine. What medication can she take? The best antidepressant in this case is Wellbutrin, which can increase norepinephrine, the precursor of dopamine.

Chemical Meltdown

What happens when brain chemicals are so messed up that self-destruction seems to be the only solution? Total hormonal deterioration, a chemical meltdown of sorts, can lead to wide-ranging avoidance behaviors, irrational fears and a dissociative personality. This means that the person falls apart and considers death as an option. A letter I received from Alex, a flight attendant in Australia, tells her story.

"Dear doctor," Alex wrote. "I have feelings of emptiness and use-lessness, although I am told how capable and intelligent I am. 'You're so beautiful; you have a great body, you're so lucky to have accomplished more than others.' I hear this all the time. I recently lost my job with an airline (one of only two in Australia) after it went broke. Thousands lost their jobs and my relationship with a great guy, who lives on the other side of the country, ended because it was no longer easy for me to visit him on my flights with my job."

"I had to rent my house out as I couldn't afford the mortgage repayments and now I'm living with my mother, I went to France to try and work on the mega-yachts but stayed only three weeks as my head wasn't there. I cried every night, came back to Perth and have been depressed ever since. I have no self worth and constantly think of ending it all. I don't see anything positive in my future. I am aging and people can't believe my age. I can't seem to shake off these feelings."

Alex blames her age and the loss of her job as a cause of her depression. She has no idea that her feelings are related to chemicals in her brain. The angrier she becomes, the more her brain function degenerates and the higher her cortisol escalates from the constant stress. This translates to still more anger turned inward that can lead to high blood pressure, irregular heart rates and suicide. The impulse for suicide may be sudden and illogical. If Alex's depression remains untreated, this young lady may be at high risk for taking her life or developing some other chronic diseases associated with depression.

The loss of her job might have triggered Alex's depressive disorder. At first she may have become stressed out because of the loss of her lover and the broken relationship. Each of these factors is the reason she uses to explain her sadness and she is correct in realizing that something is wrong. The decisive conditions creating her misery involve her hormonal chaos and not her job or boyfriend problems. She is not really listening to herself.

If she did listen, what might she hear? An undertone whispering, "I have no self worth." *Thinking of ending it all* is not a rational human reaction to stress. The real tragedy would occur if Alex never told anyone else about her feelings, threatened suicide and was ignored. Suicidal threats must be taken seriously.

To function normally, your brain depends on a good supply of all its mood-altering chemicals. Either a deficiency or excess of hormones, neurotransmitters or inadequate light can lead to depression and premature death. Left untreated, depression can become so serious that the mind decides that "ending it all" is the only way out. A person who feels life is not worth living is in great danger!

> *Tip: If anyone you know threatens suicide, take them seriously and call their doctor or take them to a mental health facility.*

Tragically, suicide still occurs in up to 15 percent of depressed patients, frequently elderly men. My 55-year-old patient, George has contemplated death. Hearing his story, which is graver than Alex's, will give you a picture of what can happen.

"I have lost interest in my wife, my job, my life," George says. "They said I was depressed, but nothing has helped. I took all the antidepressants and still feel bad. I feel like there is no hope left for me. I may as well just drown my sorrows in a bottle or the river. Now the doctor says I am just getting old. I am only 55. Is this normal?"

George is in the depths of an extreme depression. He could have the unipolar variety, manifesting a constant sense of despair and hopelessness. Or, he may have another variant called "bipolar depression" with moods that swing between mania, a particularly excited state, or hypomania, a condition that causes him to feel agitated, irritable and fearful.

People with bipolar (manic-depressive) depression experience disruption of their normal day-to-night rhythm. The combination of the circadian disruption and the unbridled craze of a manic episode can be deadly. Sufferers from this type of depression commit suicide *three times* as frequently as those with unipolar depression. Many men, like George, fail to improve with standard antidepressant therapy because it is not effective. This disorder is often associated with alcohol abuse and the use of illicit drugs or a strong family history of several close relatives with the same thing.

George most likely didn't tell his doctor that he was not responding to medication because, like most men, he is not keen on talking about anything personal with his doctor. However, without help, George's mental state may deteriorate and he may end up hurting himself or self-medicating with alcohol. In other words, George will suffer and then drink to ease his pain. This is opposite to the common holiday celebration wherein people treat themselves with alcohol then suffer from the hangover.

Tip: When your spouse's drinking habits change, consider this a dangerous sign of an impending mood disorder.

Out of desperation, many depressed people turn to mood-altering drugs such as cocaine, speed or "uppers," and Valium®, sleeping pills, marijuana or downers"—all available in most big cities. Law abiding citizens often resort to legal mind-altering drugs such as alcohol, nicotine or caffeine—anything to make them feel better.

Depression runs rampant in 75 percent of all drug abusers, including alcoholics. Yet patients who have had their symptoms medically treated sometimes continue to misuse narcotics, downers, tranquilizers, or sleeping pills. When they visit their doctors, their depression has not disappeared, but they won't confide in their physician.

Without a doubt depression is more common than we once thought. This "hidden diagnosis" should be pursued aggressively if anyone is constantly complaining and acts as if they have some unknown or undiagnosed disease. Regardless of the cause, all types of depression—from "dysthymia" (constant sadness) to major depressive disorder (unipolar) or bipolar disorder—respond to antidepressants, mood stabilizers or both, in combination with other therapies such as correct hormone replacement.

Antidepressants have therapeutic value in other conditions not associated with depression. Pain disorders such as chronic pain syndrome, migraine headaches and fibromyalgia respond well to antidepressants. Irritable bowel syndrome, chronic fatigue syndrome and premenstrual syndrome can each be successfully treated with antidepressants.

Paying attention to your hormones is good preventive medicine. By taking time to treat yourself as you treat others and by reducing stress before it becomes unmanageable, you may be able to avert the onset of a major disease. By increasing exercise before the pain of inactivity sets in or by seeing an understanding physician or psychologist when you start to experience emotional problems, you can avert the disruption of your neurochemicals.

Hormones still get mixed up despite well-intentioned prescriptions for hormone therapy. Endocrine disruptive chemicals: PCBs, PVCs and dioxin can affect you as a newborn. You might not notice the effects until adulthood, but there was little you could have done to regulate your hormones.

We have hardly any control over the unwelcome transfer of hormones into our bodies. Hormonal therapy, optimally prescribed by a doctor, has turned into a tangled mess. According to Theo Colborn, senior scientist at the World Wildlife Fund, "we are neutering the population, we are making females more masculine and we are making males more feminine. We've uncovered a new series of subtle effects, which probably take place during embryonic and fetal development and which have long-term effects that keep an individual from reaching his or her full development."

To stop the disruption of your endocrine system, you must find out to what extent your vital hormones are required to keep you feeling fine. Before those levels drop, at least you will have some baseline to refer to. I strongly urge each person who reads this book to ask his or her physician for a hormone checkup.

The good news is that the vast majority of depressed persons can find complete relief from their symptoms. With several new medications, talk therapy, or a combination of both doctors can temporarily "cure" depression. In the near future, treating sadness with hormones or light therapy and possibly curing depression with CRF-blocking medicines could become a more efficient way of dealing with this all-encompassing illness.

5

A HORMONE CHECKUP

Aggression and Its Effect on Self-Esteem

Bobby is bullying younger children at school. Barry is biting his baby-sitter. Tommy is screaming at his parents because he's convinced that they're all scheming to drive him crazy. As Mary goes through her "time of the month" she is sure that everyone around her has an attitude problem. Recognize any of these people? Are they aggressive?

Aggressiveness is defined as "a generalized disposition to engage in physically combative or competitive interactions with male peers." Is this what's happening to Bobby or Barry, or are they merely developing their ego and self-confidence? The picture is considerably more complex than it may appear.

Are these examples of emotional problems or too much hormone? The answer depends on which sex hormones are at play at what point in an individual's life. During puberty, boys are expected to become more aggressive due to increases in testosterone. Girls going through puberty may show disrespectful behavior triggered by outpourings of estrogen. So is it estrogen or testosterone that causes hostility?

Sharp increases in testosterone levels can promote aggressive behavior that may include competitiveness, related to job performance, in contrast to physical and verbal aggression. These activities have been labeled "testosterone behaviors," but does that mean they are necessarily unhealthy? Sometimes aggression is associated with irritability or anger. Does that mean testosterone is the culprit? Not at all!

Competition and desire for dominance are typically associated with aggression. In this way aggressive behavior can be seen in a favorable light as an inspiration for motivation, high self-esteem and strong leadership. In men, a competitive drive for financial success is related to testosterone dominance. Research shows that younger men are more competitive than older men in a variety of areas, but they are also more physically and verbally aggressive than women. These behaviors *are* related to the higher testosterone levels commonly seen in these young men. It's true that high testosterone drives certain types of hostile behavior.

In general, men are driven to succeed by testosterone. They want to prove their manhood and believe this requires playing a dominant role in the family, workplace and society. In their desire to surpass others, a few men will turn to drugs to give them that "edge." Drugs that increase testosterone can affect your normal self-regulating system creating serious problems down the road. Higher levels of testosterone have often been blamed for physically aggressive behavior in men. In one study men using *four times* the normal dose of testosterone, reported that their aggressive feelings did *not* increase.

Contrary to common perception, this study was one of several, which seemed to point the finger at the sudden *drop in testosterone*, rather than high testosterone that results in aggressive behavior among males and females. This paradox in the interaction of hormones relies on the effect of free testosterone on the brain as it converts to estrogen. The enzyme, aromatase, encourages the rapid change of brain testosterone into estrogen. This might explain why excess testosterone acting on estrogen receptors can cause moodiness and violence.

The highest testosterone levels are found in prosecuting attorneys, actors, doctors and business executives. You probably know a few aggressive women who have succeeded in these same occupations, but their success is generally thought of as demonstrating "masculine characteristics."

Aggression has several components, which are classified as either physical or sexual. "Physical" aggression is expressed as socially acceptable conduct. It may make itself known as vigorous sexual activity among healthy young men. Physical aggression seems to correlate most closely with high estradiol levels while sexual aggression is associated more closely with high dihydrotestosterone or DHT levels. "Sexual" aggression, in contrast, is often not tolerable in social settings. Whether it is physical or sexual, aggression engages the brain in a complex interaction of hormones as DHT and estradiol both stem from the conversion of free testosterone.

Hormonal dysfunction resulting in aggression can interfere with life's basic needs. Yet, the human body is amazing in its efficiency and self-regulating ability. Accurate testing and appropriate therapies can restore normal function in the majority of men and women with hormonal deficiencies. All you have to do to do is to take the time to have your doctor check your hormones. Paying attention to your endocrine system is the first step in restoring the hormonal harmony in your life.

Why Do We Call Testosterone, "The Big T"?

"The role of testosterone in male sexual function remains complex and controversial." Still testosterone leads the parade of hormones in importance, especially for men but comes in dead last in terms of understanding by medical and non-medical persons alike. Bodybuilders like to call testosterone "The Big T" because it is such a powerful hormone and has such a huge impact on both our body and our brain. Persons with low testosterone numbers are driven to seek out solutions.

In the first chapter of this book we looked at several of the distinguishing functions of testosterone in the male, including penis and beard growth and how the penis becomes erect for sexual intercourse. Like other hormones we have discussed in this book, testosterone is a steroid hormone created by your body to perform vital tasks in regulating, stimulating and controlling your body and your brain. Similar to other fatty compounds, testosterone consists of molecules of hydrogen and carbon bound so tightly together that they shed water and dissolve only in oil or alcohol. This fact allows testosterone to enter your brain from the blood stream by crossing the blood-brain barrier.

All steroids, including DHEA androstenedione androstenediol and DHT, are variations of the same basic steroid configuration. They are *endogenous* hormones, meaning the body generates them biologically. Those steroids manufactured by molecular manipulation mimic the structure and actions of biological compounds. They are termed *exogenous* steroids because they originate outside the body.

The word "testosterone" has found its way into our everyday vocabulary because of its association with male virility and raw muscular power. Testosterone has been around for ages, but in the 1960s it was discovered by athletes looking to gain an advantage by becoming bigger, stronger and faster than their opponents. The athlete's use of testosterone rapidly deteriorated to abuse. In 1969, the exploitation lead to prohibitions by the Food and Drug Administration when the Big T was reclassified as a Class III substance. Now it is in the same category as narcotics, pain meds, sleepers and tranquilizers.

Because of its power to create manliness, muscle and motivation, testosterone is the undisputed king of the hormones. Though testosterone holds total sovereignty over men, it may currently be gaining equal status for women as well. As significant as the Big T may be, when testosterone levels are less than optimum, a man's sexual performance and confidence suffers.

Unrecognized and untreated, testosterone deficiencies cause untold physical and emotional problems for millions of Americans. The misuse of this powerful hormone has produced distressing consequences for men and women who may really need its awesome enhancement.

Diagnosing a Testosterone Deficiency (Mostly for Doctors)

"A single measurement of testosterone is not sufficient to diagnose hypogonadism," according to Dr. Adrian Dobbs, a respected endocrinologist and andrologist. For some men the optimal testosterone level is below average; for others it is above. The gray zones blend into normal ranges and nobody knows what levels is best for everyone. You, a regular guy, on the other hand, have to accept a decision based on a single sample of blood. Is there a better way?

Hypogonadism, a low level of testosterone, must be detected and treated early on to restore normal sexual function. By now you must realize that morning or nighttime erections should occur daily in a man with normal penile function. The diagnosis of hypogonadism requires an early morning blood test to check the testosterone level before starting any hormone therapy in men under 40. For the most accurate results in younger men, samples should be collected between 6 and 8 a.m. Let me give you an example of a man I treated.

Tom, a heavyset 34-year-old sales manager with two children, wrote to me about how his low libido was affecting his marriage.

"I get lots of exercise, I watch what I eat, am not depressed, get a good amount of sleep and have a satisfying job. I don't seem to have much interest in sex and have not had sex yet this year. I also feel old and tired. My lack of sexual enthusiasm is hurting my relationship with my wife. I have heard that there may be new ways to regain a more active sexuality and I would like to try."

Tom's lack of sexual enthusiasm sounds compatible with low levels of free testosterone, the major enabling ingredient. In addition, Tom could be deficient in oxytocin, which we discussed as vital for a man to climax with a strong erection and a maximum volume of ejaculate. This may not be as important to a woman but men gauge their masculinity by outrageous parameters. I treated Tom with my transdermal testosterone cream and his problems disappeared in three weeks, as his orgasms improved.

How can you find out if you have a problem with any of your internal hormones and then treat it appropriately? Let's have two doctors tell us: Mark and Phil share office space in a family practice center and one afternoon these two colleagues pause to chat about testosterone testing.

"My patient wants me to check his testosterone," says Mark, "so I'm just going to run a test to see what his total testosterone level is. That should be enough tell me if there's a deficiency, shouldn't it?"

"Not necessarily," Phil replies. "I've been reading up on this and what I'm finding is that a blood test for total testosterone (T) doesn't give a complete picture. The amount of testosterone that is actually available to the tissues (free and bioavailable) is more important, though it's only a small percentage of the total testosterone. Seems to me, we've been looking at the wrong part of the T reserve."

"Yeah, but is this extra testing worth the expense? Can't we just extrapolate?" Mark tucks his stethoscope into his coat pocket and disappears into an exam room as he mumbles, "We've always measured total T."

Phil is on the right track, but too many doctors stop where Mark did, assuming that testing total testosterone is sufficient for a diagnosis. Both Mark and Phil should be using equilibrium dialysis, a newer sensitive test that has been developed to measure "free" (or circulating) levels of testosterone (FT). Measuring hormones in saliva and blood provides a more accurate picture of what is going on. Bioavailable testosterone (BT), which travels through the blood stream carried by the protein albumen, also gives an idea of testosterone activity and it is considered the "weakly bound" testosterone, comprising about 30 percent of the total T.

A Hormone Checkup

Your doctor should measure your free testosterone because sexual desire is more closely associated with this form. At a concentration of free T that is optimum for you, you should enjoy enhanced erotic urges, experience the desire for frequent sexual activity, notice improved strength and endurance and have more sleep-related erections. The effect of total T on spontaneous erections is unclear but men with higher free T have more spontaneous erections.

Physicians, who specialize in endocrinology, order a comprehensive hormone profile checking a patient's BT, DHT or dihydrotestosterone in addition to their total testosterone (TT) levels. They will also test for the pituitary hormones such as prolactin, follicle stimulating (FSH) and luteinizing hormone (LH), plus the sex hormone binding protein known as SHBG. Primary care doctors are often too busy to do all these hormone tests. You should be getting the idea that knowing your *free hormone reading* is an important step in planning for your future sexual health. I couldn't agree more.

Testosterone increases a man's sexual drive and encourages firm, long-lasting erections. Research indicates that the frequency of ejaculation and sexual drive are each related to the amount of FT circulating in the bloodstream. Free testosterone, as measured by *equilibrium dialysis*, provides a clear-cut computation of the degree of hormonal deficiency. In females, free testosterone increases lubrication to their sexual organs and contributes to orgasmic ability. In males, two to four percent of the TT is found in the free form yet in females it's less than one percent.

Total testosterone levels could measure sexual activity, except there is such a huge variability in this hormone among the sexes. In addition, T levels can vary from hour to hour. Sometimes taking an average of *three* morning specimens, when numbers are supposed to be higher, provides more precise readings. This approach is both cumbersome and too expensive.

Analysis by Dr. Guay and his group have estimated the "average" blood levels of testosterone for the different age groups. The generally acceptable range of total testosterone values was previously between 300 and 1030 nanograms per deciliter (ng/dl) for a man and 10 to 55 ng/dl for a woman. A nanogram (ng) is one billionth of a gram and a deciliter is one hundredth of a liter. A liter is equal to about one quart. These are miniscule amounts but the new ranges are listed in Appendix B.

A more exact assessment of testosterone activity is to measure what we call the bioavailable form or BT, a fancy word for testosterone that is available to interact with the androgen receptor. In simple terms, bioavailable testosterone *includes* the free T (FT) component of human blood. About one third of the total T is bioavailable and FT comprises about two percent in men and one percent in women.

When BT reserves drop too low, symptoms ranging from loss of sexual drive to failure to reach orgasm can result. We know that measuring FT or BT provides a better estimate of how masculine hormones are functioning in the body than does the measurement of TT. Certain labs use the age-specific normal ranges of bioavailable T, which document the fact that it declines with aging.

Nonetheless, low testosterone cannot always be easily identified by a physical examination, even with a clinical profile showing the amount of testosterone in its various forms. A complete picture of the hormone interrelationship can provide a suitable diagnosis, but some medical detective work is still necessary. How can you help your husband's doctor in this matter?

All men should provide a *detailed* medical and sexual history to their physician. To help a doctor pinpoint the basis for the problem, make certain that your spouse reveals all prescription and non-prescription drugs he takes. Past drug use, family or other relationship problems, sexual difficulties and major life events and more information about the health of their immediate family members are required. How many men can produce that information? In spite of that, the doctor needs these bits and pieces as clues to make an accurate diagnosis. If your mate can't provide them, you should go to the office with him and tell the doctor what he needs to know.

General practitioners cannot refer to a simple chart on the wall to check if there is a testosterone deficiency. Hormone levels vary widely from person to person and change for each individual according to his/her age. Sexual orientation and race each play a part in the diagnosis. Asian men and women, for example, develop lower T levels as they age and African Americans have higher T levels at any age than white Europeans. Homosexual men seem to notice a testosterone shortage at a much earlier age than heterosexuals. Women observe a disappearance of their sexual dreams as T levels drop when approaching menopause, but afterwards some develop even higher testosterone and notice an *increase*d libido.

Differences in age, race, activity and sexual appetite, or prior use of hormones and drugs or alcohol can influence hormone test results. On average, male testosterone levels drop by about 110 ng/dl for *each decade* of life. By age 60, some men's levels may be more than 500 points lower than at puberty. If at all possible hormone levels should be checked at around age 35 years of age to determine a baseline for future assessment.

While detailed laboratory testing may be useful, tailored hormone replacement therapy is impossible without an accurate hormone determination. One reason is that too much hormone in the dose can completely alter its action, reversing the intended effect.

Another more common problem is the fact that men's FT levels fluctuate wildly during their lifetime. Also the "norm" for testosterone can vary significantly between individuals and at different life stages.

In my clinic I routinely test my patients to be sure they are absorbing adequate testosterone. I monitor testosterone (FT) for one to three months until levels stabilize. Then I fine-tune estrogen, T, DHT and DHEA, measuring as often as every three months by sending out early morning samples to a reputable endocrine laboratory. I recommend hormone testing for all men and women over the age of 45.

Any young man who is unable to grow a beard or a mustache and cannot develop a muscular physique after working out for years with weights could have low DHT levels. Specific penile reflexes can provide a clue to testosterone deficiency or hypogonadism. Both sexes notice less intense sexual arousal as they get older, but a man who suddenly loses his erections and starts getting "hot flashes" definitely has a hormonal problem. If during an examination he has a loss of the *cremasteric or bulbourethral reflexes*, then something is wrong. Women can start having hot flashes as early as 40 years of age but if they have had a hysterectomy or their ovaries removed, they instantly enter menopause.

Younger and younger patient with testosterone deficiency appear in my office, many of whom I refer to endocrinologists for consultation. These primary hormone specialists usually follow a course of action recommended by the American Academy of Clinical Endocrinologists (AACE) for the treatment of hypogonadism. While these guidelines give clear information about hormone replacement for any man suffering from T deficiency, most family practice doctors do not follow them and do not know that they exist. In April of 2005, testosterone guidelines were determined for women.

Guidelines recommend the kind of testing a doctor should perform when a man's testosterone is in the normal range but deficiency symptoms are present. Like Mark, the physician we overheard earlier in this chapter, many doctors are unaware of these new procedures and continue measuring total T instead of free T; telling their patients they are "normal" when they are suffering an obvious deficiency. Consequently, millions are not being properly diagnosed or treated.

Translated into plain English, the guidelines state that all men with symptoms of a testosterone deficiency should be "treated with hormone replacement therapy." These guiding principles are written for any doctor but are usually adhered to only by endocrinologists treating hypogonadism. If you are having trouble finding an endocrinologist, you can find a list by state from the AACE. These are available at: http://www.aace.com/memsearch.php.

The complete AACE standards for testosterone prescribing, published in 2003, are too complex for most non-medical people, but if you've carefully read my definitions and explanations, you may understand some of the information. You can find more at: www.aace.com/clin/guidelines/sexdysguid.pdf.

Further testing is indicated for patients with symptoms of low testosterone whose test results indicate normal levels. These patients should be retested for free testosterone, pituitary hormones and sex hormone-binding globulin levels. Any medical laboratory can perform these tests, but endocrine labs specialize in these evaluations and are better able to provide consistent, accurate and reproducible results.

The AACE guidelines do not attempt to explain why we are seeing more cases of testosterone deficiency in industrialized countries. Though numerous environmental factors have been mentioned, more research is needed in order to understand how these factors give rise to the widespread testosterone deficiency in our population.

What About Saliva Hormone Testing—Is It Accurate?

Special laboratory tests are available to pinpoint hormone deficiencies. Hormone levels can be determined with analysis of your saliva. Saliva test kits are available to anyone without prescription except in the states of New York and California. In other states hormonal levels can be accurately measured in a teaspoon-sized sample of saliva collected in the early morning.

Saliva test kits can be ordered over the Internet and are less costly than blood or serum tests for the very same hormones. These evaluations can prove marriage saving for those who cannot afford traditional blood tests. In all states blood serum tests are more commonly used for diagnosis, but their higher cost makes them unpopular with patients.

Salivary hormone testing is uncomplicated and economical. Saliva testing allows anyone to take hormone testing to a new level. But only a few medical laboratories in the United States do not require a doctor's prescription for testing using blood samples. Hormone testing labs, which perform salivary hormone testing, are listed following the appendix.

Saliva can be used to test for LH and FSH, the regulating hormones that reflect pituitary function. Benefits include the absence of any risk of disease, pain or cross infection. Minimal time and effort are required and at one-fifth the cost. Best of all, the tests can be conducted in the comfort of your home without spending time in a doctor's waiting room.

Not all doctors of medicine accept the use of saliva testing for screening and diagnosing hormone deficiencies because it is only 85 to 90 percent accurate. But appropriate therapy can make all the difference in the world for a man whose life lacks the passion that makes a sexual relationship fulfilling. Jonathan is someone who epitomizes this observation. Healthy at 50 years of age, Jonathan made an appointment with his doctor. After a physical, his doctor told him he was in perfect health, but Jonathan wanted a second opinion.

"I have been experiencing low libido in the last few years as well as low energy and I seldom experience morning or spontaneous erections. I have only a mild interest in sex, which is alarming considering my past healthy sex drive." He had mentioned these concerns to his previous doctor.

Jonathan explored possible causes and it seemed to him that hypogonadism was the logical explanation. His father told him that he had also experienced a loss of sex drive at the same age and he was aware that there could be a genetic component to this. Jonathan was motivated to find serious answers to his questions, so he came to see me.

I ran a complete battery of tests and found significant deficiencies in Jonathan's bioavailable testosterone levels. It was relatively easy, in this case, to prescribe testosterone replacement and put Jonathan back on the road to full recovery. Three months later he telephoned me at the office. "If I keep improving at this rate, I don't know what my wife is going to do. She says she wants a honeymoon before our 25th wedding anniversary this summer. She says I'm a new man."

Let me point out again that in young men values from serum or blood hormone testing are *time sensitive*. Testosterone or DHEA must be measured between 6 and 8 a.m. for significant results. Melatonin must be measured between 11 p.m. and 1 a.m. for testing to be accurate and cortisol levels should be measured at four specific times during the day to determine the pattern of secretion. If you think this is complicated, you are right. But there is an easier approach for testing hormones.

A simple early morning saliva sample can be screened for sex hormone deficiencies. Research shows that results of saliva tests match those collected from blood. Supporting research indicates that testing saliva actually provides a better measure of bioavailable testosterone than blood tests. *Most major insurance companies will pay for this form of testing.*

Multiple hormone tests are sometimes needed for a correct diagnosis, but not all medical laboratories are equipped to perform testing using saliva. Refer to the back of the book for a list of laboratories that provide accurate results.

The ideal testosterone treatment plan involves a flexible mode of T delivery that raises hormone levels in small increments while restoring sexual function. Your doctor may be concerned about the risk of prostate cancer. To help you both realize the benefits of testosterone replacement therapy in *preventing* prostate cancer some new research is presented.

The Prostate: An Important Sex Gland

Man's second most important sexual gland is the prostate. Though the prostate is important to assure sperm's reproductive capacity, this gland gets little respect from its owners. Men get squeamish when a doctor wants to insert something into them. Some men dread the prostate examination so much that they avoid going to the doctor. When they cannot urinate properly, they would rather sit down to pee than find out if a prostate problem exists.

Man-made testosterones have been used for decades without increasing the risk of prostate cancer. While the effect of their use in older men needs further study, new evidence indicates that low testosterone may be a risk factor for prostate cancer. A 24-year study in Finland involving thousands of men showed no increase in the occurrence of prostate cancer in relation to SHBG, testosterone, progesterone or androstenedione. Yet, several doctors are still reluctant to prescribe testosterone products to their older male patients for fear of triggering prostate cancer.

Another concern is prostate enlargement. Male sex hormones such as testosterone and DHT provide the primary signal for the start of cell division in a normal prostate. Unchecked, this effect could result in non-cancerous enlargement of the prostate gland, known medically as *benign prostate hyperplasia* or BPH.

BPH develops in most men as they age but it does not always become cancer. Medical evidence indicates that testosterone may block some age-related changes that promote increased growth of the prostate. The conversion of free testosterone to DHT is blamed as the primary cause of the enlargement of the prostate gland. The process of converting free testosterone to DHT within the prostate does make cells grow and multiply. Hormonal changes probably precede the enlargement of the prostate to a certain degree and so high levels of DHT have been blamed for the condition.

The prostate specific antigen (PSA) is a protein normally produced by prostate cells but manufactured in excess by cells in prostate cancers. The PSA test, approved in 1986, measures levels of prostate-specific antigen and has been credited with detecting prostate cancer in its early stages 80 percent of the time. This test can also detect an increase in volume of the prostate as occurs in benign or non-cancerous prostate enlargement. The test is not foolproof. A research team evaluated 6,691 volunteers at the Washington University School of Medicine in St. Louis, finding fewer than 60 men with prostate cancer had a "healthy" PSA reading 82 percent of the time.

A limited number of studies in 1997 by Adrian Dobs, chief endocrinologist at Johns Hopkins, found only mild increases in the PSA after administering weekly T injections for up to two years. Normal functioning of the prostate appears to depend on the balance between T and estrogen and DHT. These ratios are crucial for endocrinologists and for the FDA to evaluate the safety or effectiveness of hormone therapy.

While the PSA test misses a few prostate cancer cases, it is effective enough to justify widespread use. Because of the possible effect of testosterone on an existing prostate cancer, the physician should always perform the PSA test and a digital rectal exam before prescribing any hormone treatments for men. The size of the prostate, as determined by the physical exam or visualization by ultrasound, is usually proportional to the PSA.

Prostate cancer is still not easy to detect early and it cannot be detected with just a digital rectal exam and testing for PSA. If a physician is suspicious of a hidden prostate cancer due to a low ratio of testosterone to estrogen, a diagnostic ultrasound should be added to the screening examination.

A well-respected urologist, Wayne Meikle at University of Utah, has done important work in this field and found that using testosterone did not lead to enlarged prostate glands or prostate cancers. Family history plays a principal role in this common cancer of elderly men. The risk multiplies in men with low T levels. Men from families with a history of prostate cancer are more susceptible to it, if their circulating testosterone falls below the minimum range for their age.

Even if physicians are trained to diagnose and treat sexual diseases and disorders, many do not have an opportunity to deal with these problems. One reason is simply that men do not like to talk to their doctors or anyone else about their sexual problems because they are embarrassed.

This policy of silence creates handicaps for the doctor, the patient and the spouse. When health issues are not addressed sexual dysfunction can become permanent. Prostate infections, for example, may progress without detection, leading to infertility and impotence. Prostate infections can be painless and long lasting or chronic.

Men need to stop pretending they are invulnerable and pay attention to their prostate. Women should encourage men to obtain medical help for sexual problems and be alert to possible problems with their own sex life. Don't wait for information. Ask questions in a positive way. Be helpful and persistent. You can be a significant partner in your man's health care decisions.

Lloyd, an elderly gentleman, wrote to thank me for sending him information about prostate cancer. "It looks like I should probably get the prostate biopsy, since my father had prostate cancer, which was discovered when he was in his late seventies. He had radiation and is now fine at 85, although he might still be fine if he had done nothing." Lloyd has obviously been thinking of all the options. He continues, "It may turn out not to have been such a good thing that I've been using testosterone. On the other hand, if I do have cancer I might never have found it otherwise."

Is Lloyd correct? Does a reliable blood test for cancer exist? Various hormones are involved in the growth of the prostate and its enlargement. The problem is not simply one of too much or too little hormone. A hormonal imbalance in either direction can lead to prostate growth and the resulting problems. In addition, men with a non-malignant enlargement of the gland are statistically more likely to develop prostate cancer at a later time.

The finger points more and more to the function of estradiol, rather than to testosterone as a cancer promoter in the prostate or in breast tissue. Cancer most commonly occurs in the body of the prostate gland where estrogen acts, while DHT effects arise predominantly in the tissue lining the prostate. This leads to the theory that different concentrations of DHT in these two parts may play opposing roles in prostate growth. If this turns out to be true, testosterone could be useful in shielding men from the negative effects of estrogen excess.

Controversial research suggesting that low, rather than high testosterone may cause prostate cancer was reported over a decade ago by two highly regarded urologists, Wayne Meikle and Robert Prehn, from the Cancer Institute. Regardless of these findings, the safety of testosterone is not fully accepted. This is a subject you will want to discuss with your personal physician. According to Dr. Prehn, testosterone may protect the prostate by blocking some of the age-related changes, which promote its increased growth.

A balance of all of our hormones appears essential to maintain normal function and structure of all sexual organs, including the prostate. Both prostate and breast cancer have been linked to the presence of greater amounts of estrogen than testosterone. Researchers continue to explore this high/low testosterone paradox. Today considerable evidence suggests that DHT and E2 may be more important than testosterone in relation to prostate cancer.

The unconfirmed belief that increased prostate cancer results from testosterone restrains the prescribing habits of many doctors. As we have noted, there is no positive link between the two, but a hint that it could be is enough to dampen the prescribing of testosterone as a clinical treatment for hypogonadism.

I believe testosterone is not the villain in promoting prostate cancer that the FDA has made it out to be. In my own practice I have seen no evidence of any link between testosterone and prostate cancer and I routinely work with other physicians who agree with this hypothesis. Again, it's crucial that you review this matter with your own doctor as new studies are regularly reviewed in reputable scientific journals.

Dispelling the Myths about Testosterone

In spite of the scrutiny of modern science some "old wives' tales" live on. Testosterone replacement, for example, is surrounded by mythology that would do justice to the Dark Ages. Despite the fact that testosterone has been proven to be a safe and beneficial hormone, many doctors and their patients insist that using testosterone leads to increased aggression, prostate cancer, heart disease and hair loss. These are all false "testosterone myths."

One of the subtlest of all testosterone myths is the assumption that inability to perform sexually is part of the normal aging process. When testosterone and estrogen levels start to decline, men and women are easily distressed over losing their sexual spark or vitality. But when older men complain to their doctors about their loss of sex drive, they are often told not to worry because "it's normal."

It is *not* normal to stop having sex after age 55, nor is it normal to lose interest in sex for the duration of your older years. If your doctor tells you that your testosterone is normal, but you are having trouble with erections or orgasms, that is *not* "normal." Men who are over 40 should not assume their sexual life ends. It is a myth and a dangerous one, to believe that losing energy, muscle mass and getting fat is customary; that it's all downhill from then on. Too many positive developments in sexual medicine are occurring to justify this pessimistic view of the future.

Of course aging causes our sexual prowess to diminish slightly as do other human systems, but they should not fail prematurely. Dr. André Guay, professor of endocrinology at Harvard University, says that a 90-year-old man should be able to get an erection at least twice a week.

Not many years ago, men were referred to urologists for impotence therapy unless it was assumed that the problem was due to psychological causes. Therapy was almost primitive and the possibility of a testosterone deficiency was rarely considered. It was not until 1985, when the FDA first approved testosterone patches, that doctors seriously considered testosterone deficiency as a treatable problem. It is quite interesting to note that it often takes a pharmaceutical development to enable doctors to treat a medical condition.

That wasn't the end of confusion. For decades doctors considered total testosterone levels as the only effective screening tool to diagnose hormonal deficiency and most doctors today still go along with this outdated belief. Current research into the numerous functions of testosterone teaches us that bioavailable testosterone, not total testosterone, determines the actual amount of testosterone needed for morning erections.

The myth that testosterone deficiency is unavoidable stops many men from enjoying a vital sex life as they age. Testosterone deficiency is a multi-faceted problem associated with other hormonal inadequacies. For example, levels of oxytocin, progesterone, DHT and thyroid hormones show a parallel age-related decline to testosterone. This does not mean that we do not have a treatment.

Matt, a drummer in a rock band, suffered from a triple whammy: testosterone, DHT and thyroid deficiency. After a month of using testosterone cream and taking a thyroid replacement medication, he was feeling a lot better. "Mental clarity is still fuzzy," he said, "appetite is not great." But Matt was no longer suffering from hot flashes and sweats, felt more strength and was confident performing routine tasks "without loathing it," as he said. His libido and erections were noticeably improved. Hormones work in concert. Like many men with one deficiency, hormones originating in Matt's thyroid were also depleted.

Tip: Your doctor should recommend a complete hormone profile, as a comprehensive diagnostic tool when dealing with any sexual deficiencies.

In the past, doctors assumed that there must be something wrong with the brain of a man who complained about his sexual drive. If it wasn't psychological, perhaps tumors in the brain were sending out an excess of prolactin. You may remember that prolactin blocks the action of testosterone causing a refractory period or a break. Its purpose is to increase the length of time after sexual intercourse when a man is unable to achieve another erection. Blaming lack of libido on too much prolactin made sense, but many medical doctors still think sex problems equal brain problems.

An accurate measurement of both free and total testosterone is the first step toward helping a man with depression, memory loss and erectile dysfunction should be done prior to prescribing anything. Giving an "erection enhancer" like Viagra, or any antidepressant only treats the symptom of the disease. Traditionally, once hypogonadism has been diagnosed, the next step would be to prescribe injectable testosterone and have the patient return for monthly injections. This is not always practical.

While injections are the least expensive form of testosterone replacement, problems are associated with this approach. For example, long-term use of injectable testosterone is believed to cause increased thickness of the blood (polycythemia or erythrocytosis), liver dysfunction, fluid retention, plus elevated cholesterol levels. Other side effects may include personality disorders or prostate enlargement with difficulty in urinating. Stimulating a hidden prostate cancer is a great concern for doctors and patients alike.

Nevertheless, low-dose testosterone has been given by injection to men from 65 to 85 years of age for up to six years without any increase in the size of their prostate or the development of cancerous tissue, proving that for many men this mode of therapy is safe.

For my patients, I prefer the transdermal or skin delivery system because there are greater benefits, more individualized dose control and fewer side effects. A wide-ranging aging study in California exploded another myth that the long-term use of testosterone was dangerous. In continuing clinical trials at UCLA over six years, there was no significant increase in levels of hemoglobin, hematocrit, or the presence of sleep apnea among men using transdermal testosterone. Prostate size and PSA *did not increase*, but body weight and abdominal fat decreased significantly, while muscle strength increased-without dieting. This sounds more encouraging, doesn't it?

For decades testosterone was prescribed for chest pain or angina in men. A clinical study in 1988 shows that testosterone plays a key role in protecting men against heart disease. As I've mentioned earlier, Dr. Conrad Swartz studied hundreds of men who had heart attacks. He found that men with abnormally low levels of free testosterone had a greater risk of hardening of the arteries and that increasing their testosterone levels decreased their risk of heart attacks.

Swartz was way ahead of his time. Today heart disease is still the number one killer of Americans, but for the first time in history doctors are managing cholesterol levels with diet and cholesterol-lowering medications. Simultaneously, improved dietary habits and increased exercise have combined to result in a decline in the incidence of heart disease.

Testosterone replacement therapy (TRT) has been reevaluated by Dr. Katherine English as a treatment to help stop chest pain by expanding heart vessels as reported by the American Heart Association in 2000. Furthermore, TRT keeps supporting ligaments and tendons strong and speeds their repair. After an injury on the racetrack, a horse will be routinely treated with testosterone but the same hormone has the capability of healing humans as well. Supplemental testosterone replacement therapy has helped men heal not only their tendons but also their heart muscle. Nevertheless, in spite of overwhelming evidence as to the benefits of testosterone replacement after a heart attack or joint injury, many doctors still resist prescribing it.

Why? To this day the myth persists that a patient could have a greater risk of prostate cancer after taking supplemental testosterone. Because the prostate depends on the androgens, testosterone and DHT, to develop and maintain its various structures and functions, any cancer that develops in that organ feeds on testosterone. The concept behind the myth is that more testosterone stimulates the prostate gland raising the risk of prostate cancer. This part is simply not true.

Another study by a group of Johns Hopkins urologists looked back 15 years at men who developed prostate cancer to see if their hormones could give a clue to their development of this disease. They compared levels of free and total testosterone, sex hormone binding globulin (SHBG) and luteinizing hormone in these men, with the levels of men who did not have prostate cancer. Researchers found *no measurable differences* in these hormones among men who were destined to develop prostate cancer and those without the disease. The study proved that no predictions of prostate cancer could be made on the basis of hormone events.

A much larger Finnish survey published in 1999, collected blood from over one thousand men between the years 1968 and 1972 plus a follow-up period of 24 years. A total of 166 prostate cancer cases occurred among men who were cancer free at the beginning of the survey. No evidence was found linking levels of serum testosterone, SHBG, or androstenedione with prostate cancer in the entire study population or in the subgroups based on age or weight. The large retrospective study failed to find a cause-and-effect relationship between the concentration of the male hormone and prostate cancer.

Prostate cancer develops mostly in older men. If you think about it, adding more testosterone to the system of men with low levels of the hormone due to aging should not cause prostate cancer. If it did, wouldn't younger men whose bodies are loaded with an abundance of testosterone have the highest rate of prostate cancer? There must be some other factors involved.

Today the finger of blame for prostate cancer points to estrogen, not testosterone. Studies, including one at Tufts University, demonstrate that prostate cancer can be induced in laboratory rats by injecting them with low doses of estrogen. As men age, testosterone levels decline and the lower production does not oppose the age-related tendency to make more estrogen. Therefore estrogen levels increase in men as they age, just as testosterone levels increase in females.

For these reasons, it is essential that physicians measure both free and total testosterone levels as well as estradiol and DHT in patients who are being evaluated for hypogonadism. The type of testing performed is crucial and PSA must be included along with a rectal exam and prostate ultrasound if any signs of abnormality show up. Testosterone can make a hidden prostate cancer grow and this fear is what stops most doctors from treating men with obvious deficiency.

6

TESTOSTERONE'S ROLE IN SEX AND PENIS SIZE (FOR MEN ONLY)

Is There a Relationship Between Aging and Testosterone?

The only way you and I can avoid aging is to die before we get old. Yet some people enjoy a vigorous, fulfilling life well into their eighties, nineties and beyond. What is the reason? As you might suspect, hormones are big players in the drama of aging. The good news is that you and your doctor can manage your hormones for a pleasure-filled life in your "elder" years. All hormones diminish throughout andropause, the male equivalent of the menopause, which usually affects men 55 to 80 years of age. For women, testosterone can remain adequate throughout their menopausal years.

Testosterone is a major barometer of the aging process. As a male you enjoy your highest levels of testosterone from adolescence till about 21 to 24 years of age. From that point on, testosterone declines. At age 40, your total testosterone level begins to drop at a rate of about one percent per year. By the age of 55, your testosterone levels might be less than half what they were when you were young. At that same age, most 60 plus women who are still living will have more testosterone than you.

Lower testosterone levels affect your sex life by weakening your ability to achieve and hold a firm erection during intercourse. In addition to a weak erection, a testosterone deficiency erodes your ability to increase your lean body mass. Simply put, you won't have enough testosterone to enjoy life to its fullest, become muscular, or do it till you die.

A dramatic drop in testosterone is usually followed by weight gain and the more fat a man accumulates, the less testosterone he has. Obesity is associated not only with diabetes but also with testosterone deficiency. This is because the aromatase enzyme in your body's fat cells transforms most of your testosterone into estradiol, the most active form of estrogen. Higher estradiol (E2) levels stimulate the sex hormone binding globulin (SHBG), which binds up the small amount of testosterone remaining. SHBG thus acts like a switch turning availability of testosterone off and on.

A reduced amount of available testosterone leads to the loss of your sex drive and more estradiol increases the risk of prostate and breast cancer. Impotence is just around the corner when you begin to lose interest in sex or you don't wake up with an erection. When these signs occur in relatively young men, chemical castration from the polluted environment might be the villain. Castration, chemical or otherwise, dramatically reduces the frequency of sexual desire, masturbation and ejaculation for many men. Lifelong exposure to pesticides and environmental estrogens may also contribute to an oversupply of estrogen in its various forms.

Some men become alarmed when they feel they start losing their sexual energy and take steps to do something about it. A failure to develop an early morning erection warns men that they should tell their doctors or wives. One of my patients, Jake, a Salinas seed broker, was such a person. Jake told me that in his twenties and thirties he'd had plenty of sexual energy and led an active sex life. But by the age of 45, when we measured his total testosterone level, it was 321, down from 471 the previous year. He was quite upset because he felt he needed more testosterone. Since Jake's testosterone level had already fallen, in another 10 years it could drop well below 300 ng/dl. An estimated 20 percent of men aged 60 to 80 years complaining of low sexual energy have T levels below the normal range of 300 to 1200 ng/dl.

The amount of testosterone working in Jake's body depends on how much was bound up and therefore inactivated by the SHBG protein. Functional problems in his pituitary or his testicles could be the reason for his low total testosterone. Whatever is to blame for the disappointing sexual drive in his mid-forties, Jake can almost certainly enjoy an improved quality of life with supplemental testosterone. By bringing his levels into the middle of the normal range we may be able to slow the process.

Like Jake, many men are thrilled by the results of testosterone replacement therapy in slowing down some of the deterioration associated with aging. The physical benefits of testosterone replacement are well documented, but we need more studies on how supplementary testosterone affects moods and sex drive.

A 67-year-old man I'll call Jim, reported to me after a year and a half on AndroGel that he loved the benefits of his testosterone replacement therapy. Improvement had been gradual, but now he was hearing all sorts of affirmation. "People I haven't seen in a while have said, 'Man, have you been lifting weights or what?' My friends tell me, I'm less stressed and more patient. I don't seem to lose my temper as much as I used to. I seem to be in a better mood more often and have improved self-confidence."

As far as sex is concerned, Jim says he experiences more frequent morning erections, a fuller penis in the flaccid state and erections that seem to be harder and last longer. Sounds pretty good, but there's more:

"Something happened the other night that was pretty good," Jim said. "I was having sex with my wife and we had been at it for about 15 minutes. She had not climaxed yet. I couldn't hold back any longer, but my erection did not go away. I stayed just as hard as before. I kept going and she reached orgasm shortly thereafter, but I was amazed that I was able to continue for another10 minutes or so and she was able to climax again! I can't remember ever doing that before."

Jim was a happy man recounting a great sexual performance. What happened?

Testosterone replacement therapy improved not only his sexual drive and his moods but also shortened his recovery time after sexual intercourse.

Testosterone replacement therapy eliminates the symptoms of androgen deficiency and, over time, helps men and perhaps women too, avoid heart disease and mental deterioration. As with any long-term treatment, there are always risks to consider, but I'm sure Jim wouldn't hesitate to recommend his therapy that, at the age of 67, renewed his sexual pleasure and performance.

Do You Know Your Recovery Time?

Orgasm is always a neurohormonal response. That is, it requires both hormones and neurotransmitters to reach culmination. Dopamine and norepinephrine, the two essential neurotransmitters, are basic for nerves to communicate properly. These compounds peak with orgasm, at which point endorphins flooding the brain create feelings of pleasure and contentment. A drowsy or sedated feeling often follows. This post-orgasmic relaxation time is known as the *refractory period* and lasts from one to 8 hours for men but is far shorter for women.

The time required for a man to develop another erection after an orgasm rises with age. Young men might ejaculate as many as four times in a night but with time, this thrilling ability drops to just once each day. On the other hand, women can experience orgasm repeatedly; the frequency of their multiple orgasms is dependant on their measure of oxytocin.

The sex act is completed when the trapped blood leaves your penis after ejaculation. Your penis then becomes "flaccid" or soft. A satisfactory erection involves a five step sequence previously outlined, each driven by different hormones and neurotransmitters. Ignorance of the actual stages involved in the sexual act can occasionally lead to embarrassment. An email from a 21-year-old illustrates this confusion about what is normal or abnormal in terms of erectile function.

Michael and his girlfriend had spent a weekend of sexual pleasure, "a ton of sex," he called it, but on the second day when he went for "Round Six," he found he'd lost his steam. "I couldn't keep it hard, but the next morning I was fine and we went at it a bunch of times and then the same thing happened later that evening. I just wanted to make sure this was normal and that guys can *wear out* so to speak. I wanted to know if there was anything I can do to help shorten the recuperation time."

Michael is only 21 years old so he didn't stop to think that after six rounds of sex with a few orgasms he might need time to recuperate. During youth, the recovery time takes about an hour. Erections cannot simply be summoned into service any time a man wants to have sex. This is why Viagra, Levitra and Cialis have gained such popularity.

The appearance of the erection enhancers enabled men to control a personal medical condition that sparked a whole new attitude in the male population. Suddenly it was not as embarrassing to discuss the loss of sexual desire with their physicians, wives or partners, other men, or even the press. Bob Dole came out on television to endorse Viagra! The proliferation of articles in the lay press, as well as scientific studies in major medical journals, underscored this exploding interest.

In the past, the available treatment for loss of sexual function was limited to injections or patches of testosterone. These were not well tolerated by patients who frequently discontinued them. Viagra entered this market as an instant winner, which further drew attention to the demand for products to treat this condition. Many men with normal sexual function still use these drugs to stay hard longer or to shorten the time to resurgence so that they can enjoy sex several times in one late afternoon. That's OK! Viagra is really the first sex drug that works!

Penis Size—Does It Really Make a Difference?
(Please make sure your husband reads this.)

Testosterone directs the development of all male characteristics such as your facial and body hair, a deep voice, sexual interest and mature sperm. Normal testosterone levels guarantee the full development of your genitals from puberty to early adult life. Testosterone is so important for male sexual organ size that older men with very low levels can experience shrinking of both their testicles and penis.

In Africa, men of primitive tribes adorn and accentuate their penis rather than covering it as we do in our society. For many in our civilized society, pictures of human genitals provide visual stimulation leading to sexual arousal. A large penis is still considered a sign of increased masculinity and sexual dominance.

Judging from the load of annoying email messages coming your way, every man is yearning for a longer, fuller, larger penis. A big penis becomes either a personal possession or the primary aspect of a sexual partner. Really now, how important is penis size in experiencing a satisfying sexual relationship? According to Richard Kaye, a professor of English at Hunter College, everybody is obsessed with penis size and other physical attributes. From his piece entitled, "The Masculine Mystique," Kaye makes the following comments (used here with permission):

"At the moment, an ever-wider array of new images of the male physique permeates the culture, subjecting the body of the American male to more scrutiny than ever before as television shows like *Ally McBeal* and *The View* depict fictional and real-life women giddily discussing male performance and penis size. Are men obsessed with their penis size because they feel a woman wants it bigger?

Magazines devoted to male fitness and health seem to think so. Fitness magazines break circulation records and advertisers become bolder and bolder in selling muscular, well-hardened jocks. These magazines always say that a big penis gives women more pleasure or women admire a muscular male physique. Yet when *Playgirl* started running well-endowed male nude centerfolds, it was gay men and not women who were buying the magazine. Is there any relationship between sexual bliss and an oversized male sex organ?

So, who really cares about the size of their penis? Adolescent boys—the newest focus for worried psychologists and harried social workers, according to *The New York Times Magazine,* fret over the relative scrawniness of their physiques, worrying about the definition of their "abs" and their penis size much like young women long for ample breasts and slim waistlines. It is a democracy. Everyone has an equal right to be anxiety-ridden about his or her physique.

It does seem that men are obsessed with the size of their penis. Men with no medical deficiency in that department have somehow equated the size of their sex organ with their masculinity. The bigger their penis, the better! Men with small penises feel inadequate and wish they could enlarge it. What's your opinion?

Those men in search of a larger sex organ find questionable medical resources on the Internet for penis pumps, penis extenders or surgery to increase their penis size. They each have their place in the surplus of enhancement techniques. There must be at least a thousand companies or individuals offering some miracle product guaranteed to increase penis size by a greater dimension than seems humanly possible. Yet hundreds of thousands of men are buying products to make their penis swell. Do they work? No, none of them are effective long term, but they certainly sell well, indicating there is an enormous interest in the subject.

Two researchers reviewing the Kinsey studies on sexuality found that heterosexual men are more likely to be preoccupied with the size of their penis than are homosexual men. Penis pumps, which supposedly expand a man's penis, are a hot item in sex shops but they only engorge the penis to fill a vacuum created by the pump. Penis extenders fit over the penis so that the sexual partner feels the size. Surgery for this organ is problematic at best and is not considered medically ethical.

DHT, the primary metabolite of testosterone, is the hormone responsible for normal development of your penis and urethra, the tube that carries urine out of your body. Without enough DHT, severe malformations develop. In addition to undescended testicles and failure of penis growth, the urethra may not fuse with the penis in the womb, a condition known as hypospadias. Hypospadias has become more common than in the past, apparently due to the action of environmental estrogens neutralizing DHT action on the budding male organ.

The average penis is about 5.5 inches long and 4 inches around when erect. Your penis grows in size during various phases of fetal, childhood and adolescence. Both DHT and testosterone are responsible for the maturity of your sex organs and the maintenance of secondary sex characteristics.

These androgenic or masculinizing effects include development and maturation of your prostate, penis and the sac that holds the testicles called the *scrotum*; the development of male hair distribution such as beard, pubic, chest and armpit hair; vocal cord thickening, alterations in body musculature and fat distribution. Apart from androgens, other hormones including the growth hormone and thyroid hormone have some effect on the growth of the human penis and its eventual size.

Hypogonadism—literally, "less than normal genitals"—is a condition related to extremely low levels of testosterone that can occur in men of all ages. Depending on the age at which it strikes, hypogonadism can have life-altering effects including: abnormal penis formation, an unusually small penis, or undescended testicles in baby boys and sexual dysfunction in older men.

A penis that is less than four inches long when stretched or erect is considered to be abnormally small and is known in medical terminology as a *micropenis*. Therapy is available to correct the situation in a boy whose penis has not fully developed by puberty. Though a man with a micropenis may feel emotionally devastated, his penis could be fully functional.

At age 36, Todd was diagnosed with hypogonadism after suffering four years with fatigue, loss of libido, headaches, hot flashes, night sweats, severe loss of penis size, depression and lack of concentration. Todd's penis was always undersized. An illness as an adult caused his testicles to swell and become sensitive. He took antibiotics and the swelling and discharge went away, along with his libido. Subsequently other symptoms described above appeared. Listen to his story:

Todd wrote, "I carry all my excess weight in my abdomen and chest. I have severe loss of muscle tone and mass and a tiny penis. I fathered three children in my twenties," he said, "but my wife made comments about how my penis was small compared to that of her first husband. We finally divorced and I have since remarried. My current wife and I have had a hard time dealing with my undersize condition. She becomes distressed when we have intercourse because of my inability to get and maintain an erection. When I do achieve one she complains that she can't 'feel' me. Because of my condition our sex life is non-existent and has been extremely unsatisfactory. I have tried pills, pumps, enlarging creams and considered surgery. "

Could Todd still have low testosterone though he is obviously fertile since he has fathered children? If low testosterone during adolescence resulted in failure of his penis to develop fully, how could his fertility have remained intact?

For one thing, fertility does *not* depend on penis size. Sperm production depends on the action of estrogen and testosterone on the testicles, while the penis develops as a result of the action of DHT. Boys suffering with low DHT levels at puberty may not develop a full-sized penis and may endure sexual dysfunction later in life. Even so, these "boys" can still father children.

What's the real story? Is it possible for your penis to grow after puberty? Adolescent boys can notice a doubling of size of their penis as they approach young adulthood. Can older men experience penile growth? Fascinatingly, for men whose penis has not completed its full growth during puberty due to hypogonadism, penis growth after maturity is a reality.

Penis Growth in Adulthood

Men go to great lengths to try and increase the size of their penis. One proposed method of achieving penis growth for adult men involves applying testosterone directly to the penis. The extra testosterone is supposed to trigger the production of growth factors like IGF-1 while their free testosterone converts to DHT. The effects on the penis, if any, are not merely from local tissue expansion as occurs with a penis pump. Some men swear this works for them.

Researchers at University of California at San Francisco have found that applying testosterone directly to the genitals of boys before puberty can result in phenomenal penis growth. A study of Israeli boys with abnormally small penises—those less than 4.5 inches long when erect—using a high strength topical testosterone cream applied twice daily for several months resulted in penile enlargement. Serum DHT and free testosterone levels were measured over several months and the average penis grew 60 percent longer and 53 percent larger in diameter. Imagine the outcome if this could happen in an adult!

Frank, a patient of mine, using our 10 percent testosterone cream, shared some remarkable observations with me. "I'm still making steady progress with the topical testosterone that you had made for me," Frank wrote. "My strength has come up at least 10 pounds on every lift and my libido continues to rise. Will it continue to get better for me sexually and physically? I have fantasies now! Also, my penis is getting thicker! Six inches around! I'm very proud of my muscular accomplishments to this point. You've changed my life!

Well I've been using your T cream for almost three years now and have gained an inch in penis length and one half inch in thickness. Now my wife has a real pleasure piece."

Frank sounds like a cocky guy, but we have to wonder how much of his perceived penis augmentation is real and how much is from increased confidence. Maybe we should ask his wife. Maybe we should recheck his measurements. Six inches around, could that be correct? Can the penis really grow in adulthood?

Sure, in certain situations it is possible. Supplemental testosterone encourages gradual penile growth, once it has been converted to DHT in boys (from 11 to 16 years onward), with low testosterone levels. It does this by activating their androgen receptors in the compartments on either side of the shaft of their penis. These receptors are present and potentially responsive throughout life.

For a male to develop a normal-sized penis and a normal sex drive, androgens like testosterone and DHT are essential. That is why giving testosterone to boys soon after puberty results in rapid penile growth during adolescence; resulting in a normal-sized penis.

Until recently, medical researchers believed that the penis stopped growing during adolescence because of testosterone's final action on androgen receptors in the penis. Now we believe that these receptors may decrease after puberty but do not totally disappear. Consequently, it is possible to increase the size a man's penis at any age, if he has hypogonadism.

The age of a man plus his DHT level is the key factor in determining whether his penis can increase in size after puberty. No pill sold on the Internet is going to contain DHT, HGH or testosterone; though they may claim they contain these compounds.

A study involving boys with a growth hormone deficiency found that treatment before puberty with the human growth hormone (HGH) improved the growth of their genitals into adulthood. Following this study the question arose as to whether the penile growth was influenced by DHT, HGH or both. Researchers at UCSF Children's Medical Center concluded that androgen receptors remain sensitive to testosterone stimulation throughout adulthood.

As I have mentioned earlier, local application of testosterone cream can easily stimulate the growth of a boy's penis. Most doctors do not know this fact and go along with the consensus that penis cannot be altered except by surgery. This myth ultimately leads many grown men with small penises to feel that they were cheated by nature without realizing that potential treatments could be available to help them overcome their predicament.

My patient Brian, a local fireman, told me that though he had a normal-size penis, he was determined to use my testosterone cream to treat his low libido. A number of weeks after he began rubbing it on his scrotum he noticed a dramatic increase in the fullness and sensitivity of his penis and his testicles started to grow.

"My libido increased markedly as well," Brian told me, "so the entire experience was gratifying. Furthermore, my arthritis improved, I put on muscle like crazy and my whole sense of wellness improved. Then the gynecomastia (enlarged breasts) appeared and I freaked, stopping testosterone completely. Maybe I was taking too much, although I was simply following the prescription, except for the genital application of the cream. I can't remember what the dosage was on the applicator. I would love to get those same positive effects without the breast problem."

Brian's over-zealous use of testosterone made him feel much better, but it created excess male hormone that probably converted to estrogen. Dangerous levels of estrogen in the system are one of the most common problems faced by bodybuilders and others self-medicating with too much testosterone. Don't do this. Excess estrogen can cause problems in men as well, including sexual dysfunction, breast enlargement, aggression and moodiness. Remember, when in doubt check with your physician.

So in review, the actual length and girth of the penis depends on the action of DHT on the sex organs of a developing male. Testosterone itself governs characteristics such as increased hair and beard growth and deepening of the voice, but DHT regulates your penis dimensions, sexual drive and the growth of your prostate and testicles. Why some men's testicles swell and others shrink with testosterone cream is still a mystery. One theory is that DHT makes the testicles grow and estrogen makes them shrink. We will discuss this concept in the final chapter.

7

LIVING LONGER WITH HORMONES

Marketing Mania for a Better Life

Men and women want to live long and satisfying lives. We want to fight off the demons of old age. We want to be young and sexy forever. We all want to be able to "do it till we die." Right?

When we discuss aging, we must consider two definitions of lifespan. *Average* lifespan is the average age at which members of our species die. Improvement in average lifespan can be achieved by assuring a clean air, water and food supply. *Maximal lifespan*, or the age achieved by the longest-lived human, interests most people. Lengthening the maximal lifespan is much more difficult than increasing the average lifespan. But is it even possible?

Clever marketers watch trends and look for ways to offer eager buyers what they want. One "famous formula" weight loss program, for example, claims it can help you "drop a dress size" from size 18 to 8 in six weeks. Once you're fashionably thin, you can sign up with another company with a bosom-boosting breast cream that will help you fill a Size D cup bra in five weeks.

Then there's the "love gel" for sale that you can rub all over your skin so that your husband will be yours forever. Better yet, a special patch you can put on your penis to make it grow three inches in a month! Guaranteed!

These inducements are supported by half-truths veiled with empty promises. But they sell! For businesses with an ear tuned to the cash register, testimonials and promises are enough to turn a healthy profit. *Caching! Caching!* The booming heath and nutritional supplement industries prosper because you want a better life! But too often you don't get what you pay for.

Human Growth Hormone—Rejuvenator or False Hope?

The desire to remain young is as old as mankind. Even if eternal youth is nothing more than a faint mist on the prospect of wishful thinking, the discovery of Florida by Poncé de Léon was the result of a worldwide search for the Fountain of Youth. Many folks still believe it exists in those humid, Everglade swamplands and every winter they flock to that Southeast corner of our country. Consequently, Florida has more rejuvenation spas, compounding pharmacies and elderly folks than any other state in the Union.

Today outrageous claims attract highly educated people who should know better than to believe the impossible. Not long ago several hundred people responded to an advertisement in a bodybuilding publication for *Giant Arctic Albino Wolverine Extract*. The fact that the post office box was in rural Sweden and that there is no such thing as a giant arctic wolverine, albino or otherwise, didn't deter them. Neither did the total lack of any scientific studies nor the placement of the "advertisement" in the *humor section* of the magazine flash a warning in their minds. It may have been a joke as far as the editors were concerned, but readers were serious and wanted to know more. Could they buy it locally?

Wait, it gets more outrageous! An interviewer surveyed athletes hoping to compete in the Olympics about their willingness to consume an illegal drug if they were certain it would bring them success but it had terrible side effects. Almost everyone said they would take the drug and half of them said they'd take it for at least five years even though it could kill them. For them, life has no meaning aside from *winning*. This all-consuming drive to get the "edge" is probably as old as mankind too. Students of antiquity tell us that Greek athletes swallowed hallucinogenic mushrooms or took morphine to improve their performance. Gladiators used ephedra and other stimulating herbs before battling in front of the roaring crowds in the Roman Coliseum. Today we continue that tradition of viewing sports heroes as superstars.

Prize-winning is the name of the game for those champions who live for their sport's triumphs. Winners are separated from losers by thousandths of a second or a hundredth of a point and competitors will attempt almost anything that may maximize their performance or their size. Athletes and bodybuilders want a competitive advantage more than anything else and will take almost any supplement to boost their chances.

The dose and type of body-boosting drug athletes search for, depends on their sport and their goal. Some want to build better heart and lung performance for endurance competition. Others are looking for muscles and strength. Still others strive to compete on the basis of speed and agility. But most look for the earnings tied to success.

Whatever their desire some designer anabolic creation is waiting for them in the labs of America, promising stronger and faster bodies but guaranteed not to contain hormones or banned substances mimicking hormones.

All male sex hormones or any other anabolic substance, actual or synthetic, are considered controlled substances by the FDA and are not legally available without a prescription. That does not mean they cannot be purchased illegally on the worldwide web. Many American nutrition companies promote testosterone-boosting supplements.

Their well-documented hormonal effects (usually placebo) on motivation and physical performance are promoted. In recognition of their capability and their strength, anabolic androgenic steroids are truly potentially harmful drugs.

The pitches for these products continue to escalate worldwide. People spend billions of dollars chasing hyped-up claims that because of a twist of fate or the placebo effect; seem to provide the benefits they seek. In the end, most of them have wasted their money rarely asking the companies to fulfill their *money-back guarantee*. Companies constantly change the names and the formulas, bringing out new products to keep profits high and consumers focused on youth.

> *"Youth is a wonderful thing... what a shame to waste it on children."*   —George Bernard Shaw

Athletes represent just the tip of the iceberg for the vanity medicine industry. The huge wave of baby boomers constitutes the biggest market for supplements and anti-aging drugs. Since anti-aging is impossible, we are all going to age, this is a hoax. Everything in nature ages. Wealthy seekers of youth, who have their own personal trainers, may appear to age more slowly. But the sad truth is that all the vitamins and herbal concoctions, claiming to lengthen life, or pills and creams to increase penis and breast volume are nothing more than advertising gimmicks; no better than the snake oils of the past or the so-called anti-aging drugs of the future.

Longer Life with HGH—Myth or Reality?

An advertisement for human growth hormone reads, "If you increase your body's level of HGH, you can reverse your aging symptoms." Another marketing statement proclaims that the "benefits of higher HGH levels include moderate weight loss, increased strength, more energy, better sleep and enhanced sexual function." These advertising messages seem to be saying that HGH-based medications are the fountain of youth.

Watch out! Deception runs rampant and you need to know the facts in order to avoid being victimized by your ignorance. First of all, be aware that it is illegal to sell medically effective HGH in the US without a prescription. To get your attention, marketers claim that tiny amounts of the hormone in their product are sufficient to add muscle power and revive your sex life.

The reality is that by law, any "real" human growth hormone (HGH) in non-prescription pills or patches can be no more than the amount you would absorb from meat in an animal fed growth hormones while being fattened for the market. Though it is possible that microscopic amounts of HGH could be included in certain medicines you can buy without a prescription, they are not the same as the growth hormone your body makes. Scientists use growth hormone created through genetic manipulation of yeast cells in their research. This type of human growth hormone cannot be obtained legally without a prescription. Any manufacturer or seller who tells you their HGH pills have the same amount of human growth hormone as the HGH prescribed by a doctor is telling you an untrue story.

Another ploy for selling commercial growth hormone products on the web is the inducement that the stuff contains a hormone "releaser." The idea is that the releaser will trigger the release of therapeutic amounts of growth hormone in your body. Not true. These releaser products contain amino acids that may be part of the building blocks of human growth hormone, but they don't stimulate it. Before they can become part of the growth hormone, the amino acids must undergo a chemical transformation in the body and this change cannot occur by taking releaser pills.

Some manufacturers sell a product that claims to boost production of human growth hormone by including ingredients that raise the body's level of the insulin-like growth factor (IGF-1). Other companies claim that enzymes in their capsules or liquids stimulate the pituitary to release human growth hormone. The "enzyme" in these products is an amino acid, arginine. A shot of arginine in the vein might stimulate the pituitary to secrete a burst of growth hormone for as much as an hour, but a pill with arginine in it has no such effect. Researcher Mary Lee Vance, MD, has commented that taking a pill with arginine as an ingredient delivers as much growth hormone as eating a steak.

You may have heard of 1990 studies reported in the *New England Journal of Medicine* showing some benefits reported by 12 older men who took human growth hormone for six months. The editors of the journal state emphatically that the study was inconclusive at best and should not be used as the basis for a costly self-administered therapy with HGH.

Speaking of human growth hormone products sold on the web, Editor Jeffrey M. Dazen, a physician, is quoted as saying that "they're just a waste of money and you're better off spending your time in the gym." HGH without a prescription has been dubbed pure quackery. The millions of dollars spent on bogus human growth hormone products would be better spent on research for ways to modify the aging process. Why all the fuss about HGH? Is the stampede for human growth hormone giving positive results?

Growing Old in Spite of Anti-Aging Hormones

The aura surrounding human growth hormone (HGH) is a classic example of how unscrupulous marketers mix desire, misinformation and exaggerated claims. Middle-aged people desperate to avoid aging, though that is impossible, experiment with human growth hormone, the most advertised "anti-aging drug" on the Internet. We keep searching for anything with a promise of improved vitality, but the genuine objective of *healthy aging* is ignored.

Scientific studies demonstrate that in youth, HGH is critical for maintaining strength and vitality. Growth hormone levels decline with age but this may be due to decreases in their hormone regulators. Older adults with extremely low levels of HGH do develop flabbier midsections and weaker muscles, but so do regular folks. Conversely, only patients with true human growth deficiency, who supplement with HGH, experience a sizeable increase in lean body mass, heightened exercise performance, improved cholesterol levels or better bone density. A quick look at these benefits may lead you to the conclusion that growth hormone therapy could be an ideal way to turn back the clock. Alas, it is not so!

A researcher at Harvard Medical School conducted an experiment over 26 weeks and reported that while growth hormone seems to increase lean body mass and decrease fat in some elderly individuals, adverse effects were frequent, including diabetes, swelling and finger numbness. Until the results confirm the safety of any treatment with human growth hormone, it should be limited to controlled experimental studies in the elderly. Proper balancing of hormones looks to me as much safer than injecting anything on a daily basis.

Despite the fact that patients with a true growth hormone deficiency can develop more muscle and less fat after HGH replacement, we lack scientific proof that they will live longer or suffer less illness. Much more research is still needed and the use of growth hormone is still being investigated for its numerous "anti-aging" claims.

Like most hormones, the FDA regulates HGH. You may find advertisements about nasal sprays containing human growth hormone, but these substances contain a few micrograms, at best. They do not have enough HGH in them to come under FDA scrutiny. Not only that, but human growth hormone is such a large molecule that it cannot be absorbed through the mouth or nose. The acids in the digestive system dissolve it, making it impossible for it to perform. Only injectable growth hormone available from your pharmacy has any biological activity in the human body. Pharmaceutical grade HGH is not available in a pill or spray you can buy at the local drug store or on the net.

Several marketing companies on the Web sell capsules or liquids that allegedly stimulate the pituitary to release growth hormone.

These substances known as "secretogogues" stimulate the pituitary and other organs of the body to release precursors of HGH.

In testing for growth hormone availability, arginine is injected to stimulate its release. That makes it fit into the secretogogue category. In addition, arginine is an amino acid that synthesizes nitric oxide, the substance that regulates blood flow to the penis and vagina during sexual intercourse. But how arginine is delivered can make all the difference in the world. Arginine injected into a vein may boost a small amount of human growth hormone from the pituitary for 45 minutes or so, but an arginine capsule or tablet has no effect on growth hormone.

John Cooke, a Stanford cardiologist, invented a unique medicinal food—HeartBars™, which contained six grams of arginine in a healthy snack bar. Peripheral vascular deficiency, a condition of decreased blood flow to the legs results in pain on walking. Dr. Cooke's book, *The Cardiovascular Cure*, reveals how he fortuitously discovered that arginine had the same favorable effect on blood vessels to the heart! He demonstrated that large amounts of arginine are effective orally in increasing blood flow to our legs and arms by stimulating nitric oxide. Unither Pharma recently formulated a more advanced arginine formula, HeartBars Plus™ that dissolves in water to become a nutritious drink that can enhance circulation.

IGF-1—Mankind's Gift from Human Growth Hormone

Together we have looked at the many ways that hormones interact to keep our bodies functioning normally, but there is so much more to explore. Consider the relationship between growth, aging and eating, for instance. We are just beginning to understand some of the intricate and delicate interactions between calorie intake, growth and aging in relation to human growth hormone. We know that children eat to grow and that as they go through puberty, they need more food than at any other time of their lives.

It's all for growth. This leads us to the insulin-like growth factor known in medical circles as IGF-1. IGF-1, also called *somatomedin-C*, is not a hormone at all, but merely a molecule created in the liver that *acts like a hormone* by influencing biological activities such as growth and procreation.

A powerful molecule, IGF-1 sets changes in motion right at puberty. By attaching to muscle cells, it increases their size, not by metabolizing more protein as testosterones does, but by acting directly on the cells. IGF-1 regulates cell death, tooth development and hair growth, acting just like a hormone or as a regulating protein. Technically speaking, IGF-1 is a vital component that is taking center stage in medical research projects seeking to explain the aging process

The studies confirm that IGF-I acts on the pituitary by *inhibiting* growth hormone. The regulation of growth hormone by IGF-1 probably reflects a negative feedback loop essential for maintaining tight control over growth hormone cell function. Additional findings indicate that IGF-1 has *potent* effects in regulating growth hormone. Around the age of three, children have higher levels than before and by the age of 10 to 12 they reach adult levels. A high concentration of the IGF-1 at puberty encourages sexual maturity. In clinical studies, girls at all age levels have been found to have higher amounts of IGF-1 than boys of the same age, perhaps explaining why girls mature earlier.

After adolescence, you lose the greater part of IGF-1 circulating in your bloodstream and ultimately reach depleted levels in your old age. There is a decrease in the growth hormone releasing hormone (GHRH) and an increase in *somatostatin*. Somatostatin stops IGF-1, which blocks the action of growth hormone. A decline of these hormones is due to the altered hypothalamic regulation of ordinary aging. Again you can see how complex our endocrine system can appear, but if you pay attention you can learn that there are ways to bring your hormones into balance.

Aging is therefore the primary instigator of declining growth hor-

hormones change as you age. For example, your pi-
___ releases less and less growth hormone after you become
___its during the event named "the somatopause." This stems from
several factors that contribute to the age-related decline in growth
hormone secretion. Tests of aging men show that growth hormone
secretion declines by 50 percent every seven years after age 35 years.
Is this true aging or is it created by a disease state?

The somatopause—name some of the classic signs of aging—less
exercise, poor sleep and low sex hormones and you have the explanation for the low GH. Your growth hormone (GH) is altered by your
weight, your testosterone or estrogen and your decreased physical fitness. Because GH secretion occurs predominantly during slow-wave
sleep, levels of this hormone are modified by abnormal sleep patterns.
You know that declining levels of IGF-I along with low growth hormone are part of aging; it seems therefore that somatopause is part of
becoming old rather than a disease.

The manipulation of hormones and genes to *slow how quickly you
grow old* may one day lead to amazing outcomes in the field of longevity. But a much simpler method to add years of health to your life
already exists. What's the secret? We have covered over 200 pages to
find the best answer.

How to Slow the Aging Process

Eat Less—grow old more slowly! There it is! Experts, who study
the field of aging, gerontology, suggest cutting your daily calorie load
to about 1000 to 1200 for women and about 1500 to 1750 for men
slows deterioration. Before you conclude that semi-starvation may
not be the most expedient way to live longer, consider the following:
it works for animals, prisoners of war and an isolated group of Japanese. On the island of Okinawa, there are more centenarians, those
who live to be 100, than anywhere else on earth.

By reducing the number of calories consumed, lifespan enhancement was reported in all rodents, flies, fish and worms, as early as 1935. Laboratory rats and squirrel monkeys under caloric restriction age more slowly. In humans, only observational studies are available. Those Japanese living on Okinawa "have a forty-fold increase in odds of becoming centenarians," according to Chris Vojta, a fellow at the Institute on Aging, at the University of Pennsylvania. Andrew Weil found these ancients to be spry, eating a low-calorie diet, cheerful and mentally sharp when he visited their island. Dr. Bradley Willcox, a gerontologist from Harvard and co-investigator of the 25 year Okinawa Centenarian Study teamed up with his identical twin, Craig, a medical anthropologist and Dr. Makoto Suzuki from Okinawa University to write *The Okinawa Program*. They learned their secrets to healthy longevity and describe 16 ways to eliminate excess calories.

It could be as straightforward as this: fewer calories mean lower levels of your circulating blood sugar, insulin and lower cholesterol. This effect produces a decreased rate of cell division and free radical damage plus a lower fat mass and a more robust immune system may be responsible for this effect. Diets, including vegan (plant-based) proteins, reduce elevated cholesterol levels and decrease circulating levels of the insulin-like growth factor activity lengthening both the average and maximal lifespan.

In fact, vegans have lower blood fats, leaner physiques, slower maturation as children and a decreased risk for certain prominent "Western" cancers; a vegan diet has documented effectiveness in rheumatoid arthritis. Low-fat vegan diets may be especially protective in regard to cancers linked to insulin resistance, namely breast and colon cancer or prostate cancer. However, according to Dr. Vojta, "the long-term effect of decreases in body temperature, metabolic rate and the size of most major organs are still unknown." These are typical in those who are vegans from birth.

No positive association has yet been established between levels of the insulin-like growth factor and muscular strength, body composition and physical functioning. To explain this, scientists consider the possibility that the insulin-like growth factor levels do not really reflect growth hormone status or that they do not correlate with the biological activity of IGF-1. Before you sign up for these supplements, you should know that there isn't enough evidence to show whether treatment with IGF-1 can either slow or reverse age-related changes in human beings. Ironically, one may accelerate their death rather than turn back the hands of time if someone embarks on an unsupervised hormone-replacement program. Be careful!

It's a different story with insulin-like growth factor when we are young. Testosterone, which stimulates growth of the bones at puberty, cannot make bones grow unless there are high levels of IGF-1 present. This growth factor is thus largely responsible for the growth spurt we see at puberty. Adding three, four, five or more inches in a year is not uncommon for adolescents.

Pygmies, in contrast, grow to adulthood without achieving normal height as achieved by the majority of humans. Studies of pygmies show that they have only one-third the amount of IGF-1 compared to adults of normal height, though their levels of testosterone and human growth hormone are equal to those of normal adults. Their bodies simply stop growing at the height they reach at puberty.

Does this mean that we should consider prescribing the insulin-like growth factor to prolong life or increase height? No! The role of the IGF-1 axis in growth control and cancer promotion has recently been established at the University of Pennsylvania by the finding of elevated IGF-1 levels in association with three of the most prevalent cancers in the United States: prostate cancer, colorectal cancer and lung cancer. Lower levels of the insulin-like growth factor associated with aging may thus prove beneficial, actually inhibiting cancer induction.

In a controlled study of healthy older men and women, those taking growth hormone noticed increased lean mass and decreased fat mass. When sex steroids such as testosterone and DHT were added, increased muscle strength and lung capacity were noted in men, but not in women. These trials indicate that more research is needed before growth hormone is routinely used to attempt to delay aging or increase endurance.

Another matter for concern is the potential misuse of our healthcare resources. Growth hormone replacement for growth hormone-deficient adults with pituitary disease is expensive, costing up to ten thousand dollars a year. We do not know precisely how much growth hormone is prescribed for "off label" uses, but estimates suggest that one third of prescriptions for growth hormone in the United States are for indications for which it is not approved by the Food and Drug Administration.

I should emphasize that growth hormone therapy is *not an accepted standard of medical care* for conditions other than growth hormone deficiency though anti-aging doctors who may profit from its sales to their patients are promoting it. Growth hormone is just one hormone released from the pituitary that declines with increasing age.

This observation, together with the changes in body composition associated with adult growth hormone deficiency, has led to the suggestion by some in the "anti-aging movement" that all elderly people are deficient in growth hormone and may benefit from human growth hormone therapy. These health care professionals should also tell their patients that injecting human growth hormone just increases both estrogen and testosterone levels.

In summary, taking extra human growth hormone by injection may be a proven, safe therapy for children and adults who are markedly deficient in the hormone. Until studies prove its value in elderly persons, a better course would be to enjoy the benefits of natural growth hormone with exercise, nutrition and restful sleep. Exercise that induces sweating and rapid heart rates for short bursts of time has been scientifically proven to increase longevity.

Take the time to check your hormones, ask for testing by your doctor and request replacement therapy with testosterone, DHEA, estrogen, progesterone, melatonin or whatever hormone is found deficient after testing. This is the safest and most sensible approach to treating the ravages of time.

Should Aging Be Treated as a Disease?

So far the mortality rate of the human race is running at 100 percent, but that doesn't mean we have to look forward to our final years in the throes of pain and disease. At the close of the century there were 77,000 people 100 years or older in the US and statisticians predicted that the number of centenarians is expected to double with each decade for the foreseeable future.

Since certain hormones decline with the aging process, it is only logical to assume that hormone restoration should slow the aging process. Total testosterone, for example, declines at the rate of 110 nanograms per deciliter each year after age 40. Levels of bioavailable testosterone fall off even faster. Binding to the sex hormone binding globulin (SHBG) speeds up with aging, decreasing the amounts of free testosterone.

Healthy men and women with low testosterone enjoy a positive physical and mental effect when testosterone is administered; a leaner body, stronger muscles, better brain function and a heightened sexual drive result. Therefore it seems reasonable to incorporate hormone replacement therapy when low levels exist.

Little is known about the effectiveness of products that are being promoted to consumers as "anti-aging" therapies. Hormones decline with aging, but that does not prove that replacing them to normal levels will reverse the aging process. Such conclusions are only hypothetical and need to be substantiated by large-scale controlled clinical trials before being accepted as standard of care.

Your primary care physician should offer healthy aging as nothing more or less than the practice of good medicine. Your doctor knows that diet and moderate exercise are the essential building blocks of a healthy body and that the best source of nutrients is a balanced diet, although some older patients may benefit from Vitamins C, A, D, E or phytonutrients from organic fruits and vegetables.

As pointed out earlier, in laboratory tests a low-calorie-diet doubles and triples the lifespan of simple creatures like earthworms and fruit flies. In more sophisticated animals such as mice, monkeys and dogs, decreasing calories increases the lifespan less dramatically but these animals are being observed in a laboratory setting. Those who consume fewer calories appear to build up less resistance to insulin and increase their supply of DHEA. While it is not a wonder drug, DHEA has beneficial effects on the function of the heart, the brain and the immune system.

Is it calories, hormones, lifestyle, or exercise that makes some people age better than others? The answer may surprise you. The ability to maintain active and independent lifestyles for as long as possible is almost certainly not related to medical care, diets or hormones. When centenarians are studied for the secrets of their good health, the most important factor contributing to their longevity is always genetics. Investigators studying the lifespan have concluded that up to 35 percent of the variation in lifespan is due to genetics.

These "Methuselah" patients simply had long-lived relatives and healthy families. Most of them also refrained from the use of alcohol and tobacco. Assume for a moment that lucky genes are the sole reason for a long and healthy life. What influences these genetic factors? The answer, of course is our hormones.

Since the decoding of the human genome in 2003, mankind has come one step closer to determining the genetic factors that may one day unlock secrets of the aging process. The future may yield new medical techniques for modifying genes and slowing the aging process. The best way to guarantee a long and healthy life is by choosing parents with exemplary health. Nevertheless there are realistic steps you can take at whatever age you may be. Meanwhile we know that quality of life is much more important than quantity. Finding life pleasurable involves the enjoyment of sex, hobbies, friends, relatives and the avoidance of disease and infirmity.

In his book, *The Evolution of Aging,* Theodore Goldsmith observes that while there are reports that people who engage in sex more often live longer, it has not been established that there is a cause-and-effect relationship. After all, we can assume that people who are healthy will have a more active sex life than those who are not. Still, the increase in hormonal activity triggered by sexual relations could be a contributing feature to longevity.

Medical science will continue its fascination with the human genome and the secrets it has yet to reveal. Hormone replacement therapies will transform over time and many more uses will be found for them. Aging is still a biological phenomenon. It's a bad idea to treat aging as a disease. I prefer to put off the ravages of time by restoring health to optimum levels. This is simply good Preventive Medicine.

You can follow preventive guidelines to help avoid disease, stay alert and incorporate positive lifestyle changes. You can adopt a healthier lifestyle by giving up cigarettes and drinking alcoholic beverages only with meals. Eating more nutritional food, chewing it slowly and avoiding the use of illicit drugs will improve wellness. These simple steps won't guarantee you a long and active life, but they are essential in building a healthy mind and body for your final years.

When we look at problems associated with aging in our society, we can see that adopting wholesome strategies would reduce costs plus pain and suffering. An increase in the quality of life of the elderly enables them to remain productive and to contribute to the well-being of society. In light of these facts, public awareness needs to be increased and basic research in slowing aging should be intensified.

So why do we suffer from such dreaded fear of aging? After all, aging is a natural phenomenon, not a disease. Many folks in their eighties are still totally competent and physically functional. *Vintage People,* written by Dr. Jerry Old, celebrates the successful lives of many Americans, with stories of remarkable people in their nineties who maintain a vigorous and upbeat lifestyle. Healthy aging should be the goal of all people over the age of 65. (See www.healthyaging. com)

How Nutrients Affect Aging

Yes, we all get old, *if we're able to survive* the stress of living in a fast-paced world. But have you ever wondered why some people age gracefully with a sharp mind and physical fitness while others become crippled and lose their memory?

Nutrition might be an important reason why some get along better than others in their advancing years. In elderly patients for whom nutrition may be a problem, measurement of zinc levels is of great consequence. Zinc has an anti-aromatase action and can be used to treat low T levels. Older people can become deficient in essential vitamins such as A, C, E and D and key minerals such as calcium, zinc, magnesium, iron, chromium and selenium. Enzymes like Co-enzyme Q10 and gingko, ginseng and grapeseed have all been used as anti-aging therapies. According to nutrition expert Dr. Dean Ornish, eating fruits, vegetables and grains—a plant-based diet, will provide all these substances while avoiding excess animal proteins that are bad for the heart.

While most of your body's functions continue to operate into old age at almost 75 percent of their youthful level, your digestive system doesn't fare that well. As you age, your taste buds, the strength of your stomach acid, your thirst sensitivity and your elimination system become far less efficient. As a result, you do not absorb all the vitamins and other nutrients you eat. You have to take extra steps to be sure you incorporate enough of these valuable substances into your bodies. Many people complain about taking pills but swallow dozens of vitamins daily. There must be an easier way to get all the nutrients you need for optimum health.

With aging, your hormones gradually lose their ability to deliver their marvelous benefits. It works like this. As you grow older, you accumulate more fat and less muscle. Your kidneys don't eliminate toxic substances as efficiently and your liver loses some of its filtering capability. Altogether these factors add up to a less effective transport system for the hormones that you need to circulate freely through your body for the best of health.

Of course, not all elderly people respond identically to hormones or nutrients. Assimilation can be affected by over-the-counter medications like antihistamines or antacids that interfere with absorption. Drug-to-drug or drug-to-food interactions further contribute to problems that arise in the improper dosing and use of medications in the elderly.

Another problem with hormones used by older people is that over time the human body manufactures less of the proteins that bind to medications. Drugs that are not bound up with blood proteins reach higher than desired levels in the bloodstream. The opposite effect occurs with hormones because sex hormone binding globulin increases with aging, lowering the amount of available hormones.

With declining hormones, seniors may become dehydrated without being thirsty, malnourished without feeling hungry or constipated without being aware of an urge to have a bowel movement. These changes greatly affect the quality of their lives. Moods, appetite, energy and the absorption of medications are all affected by the passing years and your hormones.

What About Sex after 70?

There are plenty of misconceptions about aging. We do know that aging is much more complex than a simple hormone deficiency. We also know that the best defensive medicine starts with talking to your doctor about nutrition, stress reduction and enjoyable sexual communication with your partner. Be sure to ask your doctor about any problems you or your mate has with your sex life. It may not be easy because these conflicts are often masked by other disorders. In addition, many patients have difficulty discussing these personal problems openly. Regardless of your age, make the effort to be open about *all* matters related to your sexual experience.

Many Americans still think that losing their sex drive is a regular part of growing old. We expect sexual function in older Americans to decrease as they age until sooner or later sex becomes nothing more than a memory. The truth is you don't have to give up sex even if you're past 70.

Plummeting hormone levels and reduced sexual activity lead to decreased sexual interest that may be related to the aging process, but they do not completely account for age-related changes in sexuality. Your doctor must consider all the aspects of your emotional and physical health before concluding that aging is to blame for a lack of sexual interest. Stress, anger, debilitating diseases and many other conditions sometimes make their presence first known through a loss of sexual desire.

Sexual activity helps us cope with stress. The discharge of "natural opiates" plus the bonding that come with a positive sexual experience brings a touch of peace into our sometime chaotic lives. But healthy sexual functioning requires both an adequate hormonal balance plus appropriate neurotransmitter levels.

The reality is that sexual passion, physical enjoyment, a normal sex drive and thoughts of love are more important in overall life satisfaction than erections or the physical performance of the sex act. Most men consider the physical act of making love a sign of their virility instead of a form of communicating love. Women are much more sensitive to this process as they get caught up with the emotional aspects of sex. This is not always easy without an understanding partner. Women, in fact, suffer from sexual dysfunction more than men but they are more likely to discuss it with their doctors.

Hormone deficiencies are an unfortunate aspect of growing older, but by taking steps to improve your hormonal balance and discussing these problems with your personal physician, you can function at optimal balance well into your golden years. It helps to stay flexible for exercise will make you feel more sexual, but without adequate hormones, you simply go through the moves. You should be able to enjoy sex for the rest of your life.

Memory and Intelligence—the Hormones in Your Brain

High cortisol levels and sleep deprivation can both alter your moods and erode your short-term memory. Back in Chapter Three, we looked at how melatonin, regulated by light, triggers sleep and adjusts our body's rhythms. Years of research by Dr. Axel Stieger at the Max Planck Institute in Germany have shown that the growth hormone-releasing hormone, (GHRH) and the corticotropin releasing-hormone (CRF) also participate in sleep regulation and the increased retention of memory.

The growth hormone-releasing hormone works by regulating the release of growth hormone to the body during the night. Deep, dream-filled, slow wave sleep (REM sleep) is essential for its function. REM sleep is crucial for normal memory and good health and the avoidance of depression. Hormones including growth hormone, prolactin, cortisol, estradiol and melatonin blend into this complex balance to induce refreshing sleep. As just noted, raised levels of cortisol impair sleep while GHRH enhances the slow wave sleep by increasing growth hormone. Please note that hormones can antagonize each other in addition to providing balance for the best possible function.

In a study involving healthy volunteers, GHRH increased slow wave sleep (REM) and growth hormone secretion while blunting cortisol release. The combination of these effects tends to de-stress an individual during sleep allowing the brain to retain and store complex memories. Dreaming can be thought of as a descrambling process wherein blips and bleeps of memory bits are organized into some type of story. Normal sleep requires a balance of brain hormones to promote dream retention and improve memory while stimulating weight loss by lowering cortisol.

An entire new class of memory drugs is being developed to take advantage of this research. Antidepressants based on cortisol-releasing hormone blockers will reverse the cortisol excess that is so destructive in the body and the brain. Cortisol is toxic to memory cells. Agents that have a dual action, affecting both serotonin and norepinephrine are being perfected as sleep-inducing pills and antidepressants. Memory enhancing drugs that block specific enzymes are also being developed to treat Alzheimer's disease. Can anything else be done to "slow down aging" and maintain our hormonal balance?

Yes, but its not exciting or earth-shattering news. It comes down to a good diet and exercise. The growth hormone inhibitor somatostatin can be *blocked* with a healthy diet containing adequate amounts of arginine, ornithine, glutamine and other essential amino acids. You won't find these nutrients listed on the ingredient list because they are common protein components found in plants. Plants have evolved with humans to provide all the essential nutrients needed for optimal health.

Watching the amount of food you eat and decreasing IGF-1 with calorie restriction, stimulates DHEA in addition to reducing cortisol production. Besides this, pregnenolone used as a food supplement may improve memory. Hence listening to your doctor and getting the right advice is critical.

The preventive approach is simple: a healthy diet coupled with regular, moderately intense exercise (up to 65% of your maximum heart rate) increases the helpful growth hormone during the night and decreases the release of bad cortisol. A good night's sleep guarantees improved mental functioning and better weight control.

So grandma was right, "...eat your veggies, work hard at chores and get a good night's sleep and you are set to go."

Why You Should Modify Your Food Choices

The dramatic rise in youngsters who are hyperactive or suffer from Attention Deficit Disorder is a puzzle begging to be solved. Christine Wood, MD, a pediatrician and author of *How to Get Kids to Eat Great!* says we need look no further than the food our children are eating. She cites more than a dozen studies showing that when children with behavior problems eat less sugar and fewer refined foods, they are able to concentrate better and experience far fewer incidents of disruptive behavior.

It may seem like a leap of faith to link mood disorders in our children with their diet, but Neurophysiologist William Calvin in his book, *How Brains Think,* gives his perspective on how our brain developed intelligence and why we eat the way we do. Calvin feels that our ancestors led the way in adopting "basic searching moves" because they had to become omnivores and "…switch between many different food sources. They need more sensory templates (patterns), mental search images of things such as foods and the predators for which they are on the lookout." So our diets shaped our mental processes and these days, they shape much more.

By matching these mental images with the behavior required to obtain the food they were seeking, our human ancestors were able to adapt to their world. As children we pretty much eat what our parents feed us until we're old enough to forage for food on our own. All mammals go through a period as playful juveniles to learn the skills they need to survive as adults. For apes and humans this learning time is much longer and aids in the development of greater intelligence. As soon as we're old enough to make our own choices, we modify our food choices and try new things to eat. Calvin points out that a long life promotes versatility and adaptation to change by giving us more opportunities to discover new behaviors and adapt to them.

Family eating patterns help mold our likes and dislikes and either prolong or shorten our lives. Another advantage to a long life is that the longer we live, the more we can use our intelligence for our own benefit and enjoyment. This equips us with brainpower we can use to choose a calorie-reduced, toxin-avoiding, plant-based diet as a means of slowing the process of aging and the deterioration of our brains. Recognizing that a low-fat diet of whole foods can cut the harmful effects of dioxin, we can make the choices that bring our behavior into harmony with our knowledge and prolong our vitality. An active social life also prolongs life.

For most of us, a meal shared with others is more rewarding. The reality is that eating gives human beings a welcome opportunity for social interaction. As we observe what other people are eating and how they relate to their food, we have new chances to follow their example and take advantage of useful discoveries they have made. You might never enjoy peanut butter on a stalk of celery, for example, if you didn't see your father-in-law enjoying this treat. Fried green tomatoes, onion-seasoned popcorn, or muffins smothered in pizza sauce may not sound appetizing until you taste a sample at a social gathering of some kind.

We know intuitively that food is essential for life. A newborn baby has no way to avoid starving to death without a nursing mother and the infant turns instinctively to its mother for all the nutrients needed to survive and grow. If the mother of the newborn is not able to supply milk from her breast, baby formulas have been developed in an attempt by the food industry to match the nutritious value of breast milk. The reality is that while packaged baby food may contain the required amount of carbohydrates, fat, protein and vitamins, only human milk contains the antibodies essential to establish a strong immune system in the baby. Not only that, but prepared foods introduce the infant to environmental pollutants and harmful additives converting it to processed food. Most baby foods are simply ground-up adult food mixed with lots of sugar and salt.

Like the animals of the plains or the jungle, humans are always on the lookout for food. Ironically, the search is the problem because food is all over the place in America. Close by is the corner market or a super-market loaded with thousands of brands, not to mention ice cream shops, restaurants and vending machines. We have an abundance of groceries of every type and description, far more than we need. Worse, most of it is loaded with fat, sugar and more protein than we require. Food companies know that people are highly susceptible to food-related advertising in the mass media. They spend more than seven billion dollars a year telling us what they'd like us to eat. Of course we don't have to eat everything we see on television nor in restaurants. If at all possible you should not let commercial messages paid for by manufacturers of processed foodstuff determine what you eat.

Obesity is a serious problem in our society and treatment is complex. We should make our own food choices using the intelligence we have developed over the centuries and stop giving into the constant temptation. Today, as physicians we worry more about obesity killing our patients rather than having them starve to death. The need to treat overweight persons and their response is dependent on the patient's willingness to receive therapy plus their ability to comply with the doctor's recommendations.

Dr. Andrew Weil, nutrition guru at the University of Arizona Program in Integrative Medicine, made the cover of *Time Magazine* in October 2005. He was looking for the optimum diet for a given person that minimizes risks of disease and promotes health and longevity. What follows is a portion of what Dr. Weil wrote at the start of the year "A call to action by the First Annual Conference on Nutrition and Health" in a new medical journal called *Explore.*

"We believe that the population of North America is in great nutritional peril. People are consuming increasing amounts of low-quality foods. There is an epidemic of obesity and in its wake, rising incidence of type 2 diabetes in young and younger children. More people than ever are following extreme and fad diets that may pose long-term risks to health. The food served in schools, hospitals, and senior facilities promotes obesity, chronic inflammation, and accelerated development of age-related diseases. We are also concerned about food safety, given the practices of factory farming, conventional agriculture, and the genetic modification of foods. And we are dismayed to watch the successful exportation of our unhealthy foods and eating habits all over the world."

As we become more advanced about food's effect on our lifelong health and our environment, we are learning to rely less on animal fat and more on whole grains, fruits and vegetable. We should all modify our food choices based on good information and stop absorbing the advertising messages of the processed food industry. Did you know that "fast food" is addicting? Slow food, on the other hand, is healthy. Jane Goodall, the primatologist, writes about slow food diet in her new book, *Harvest for Hope : A Guide to Mindful Eating.*

Eat "junk food" and you end up with a junkyard for a body.

"Progress comes from the intelligent use of experience."
—Elbert Hubbard

The Quest for Long Life

You may want to live well into your eighties and nineties or beyond, but you probably wouldn't choose long life unless good health came with it. No doubt you would prefer to remain active and healthy while also enjoying the pleasures of youth along with the rewards of maturity.

Anti-aging has become a huge industry and is growing rapidly, but it is a folly. Thousands of products and treatments are offered today to slow the aging process. Costly anti-aging medications have emerged in the marketplace to give people the illusion that they can buy longevity—if they have enough money. They are assured that by injecting themselves every day with a human-like growth hormone, they will enjoy longer life. Not true!

Even without miracle hormones, we are already living longer than our forefathers. The elderly population is growing so fast that before long they'll be the majority. For 30 years, starting in 1970, life expectancy worldwide grew four months for each year. New forecasts project that halfway through the 21st century, the median life expectancy will surpass previous estimates by 1.3 to 8.0 years.

The over-65 population will increase by 82 percent from 2000 to 2025, although the birth rate will increase by only three percent, the world population may actually decline in the foreseeable future, with a higher percentage of individuals in their older years. Imagine the impact this will have on the global economy.

Citizens of the seven most highly developed countries (G-7) will live to the following ages, on average, by 2050:

Canada	85.26 years
France	87.81 years
Germany	83.12 years
Italy	86.26 years
Japan	90.91 years
UK	83.79 years
US	82.91 years

Notice, the US comes in dead last. Nonetheless, a projected lifespan of nearly 83 years of age by the mid 21st century, is a big jump from an average lifespan of 57 years, at the beginning of the 20th century. The number of people reaching the century mark should assure all of us that we all have the potential to live long lives.

The oldest documented human, in recent times, is a 122-year-old French woman, alive during the days of the French Revolution, who smoked and drank during the last 20 years of her life. Did smoking and drinking enhance her longevity? Not at all! Studies of centenarians have one factor in common—a genetic trait. They all had long-lived grandparents, brothers and other family members. *Genetics is the secret to long life.* You, too, could live to be 100, if you could choose your relatives.

Experts believe that the maximum possible lifespan for humans may be as long as 150 years. In the future humans may be able to live closer to their maximum lifespan thanks to genetic engineering, a more abundant supply of organs for transplantation and medical discoveries that will make replacement parts common. With such a long lifespan, people may choose to retire at age 100. The difficulty in surviving will no longer be avoiding chronic diseases, but living for more than a century without being bored.

We aren't there yet, but we do know that with advancing age, production of certain hormones declines, including human growth hormone, DHEA, oxytocin, melatonin and, of particular interest, testosterone. We have to ask: Is the decline of these hormones a normal consequence of aging, or are we dying prematurely?

The manipulation of hormones to slow the aging process could lead to amazing strides in the road to greater longevity. In the last chapter we discussed the promise of growth hormone supplements as an anti-aging agent, only to reach the conclusion that low levels of HGH and IGF-1 are healthier than high ones. The addition of specific antioxidants plus the use of sun block to minimize the photo aging of the skin is all we can do to avoid looking old, short of cosmetic surgery or laser skin resurfacing.

Meanwhile my experience in administering growth hormone to elderly people who are seriously deficient in this hormone has been remarkable. I have seen those patients enjoy improved heart function, decreased pain and weakness, better motivation and more pleasure in living. Therapy with small amounts of human growth hormone can be rejuvenating in certain people. This is different from pushing growth hormone levels into abnormal ranges and risking serious side effects for anyone who wants to "stop aging."

In the 1800s Voltaire said, "Doctors are men who prescribe medications of which they know little, to cure diseases of which they know less, in human beings of whom they know nothing." We have come a long way since then in achieving medical breakthroughs, but we have much to learn. We are still on the frontier of knowledge about many areas of health, especially regarding sleep and aging. New discoveries about how light and food can affect the changing human condition are coming in the future.

Restful sleep is essential for the best possible function of our brains. During sleep our brains and bodies recharge, providing energy for daily tasks and formatting a retentive memory to allow us to accomplish all we want. It's the lack of refreshing sleep and lower levels of the GHRH that exhaust us, as we grow old. That doesn't stop the parade of "anti-aging" and non-addicting sleep drugs.

I am continually amazed by the variety of drugs you can purchase on the Internet without a prescription. Marketers promote: both HGH and IGF-1 as magic steroids you can simply spray up your nose, melatonin-free sleeping pills, energy capsules, Leptoprin™ appetite suppressants, the list goes on and on. Do they work, or are these a cruel hoax thrust upon an unwary populace looking for more a quick fix?

8

ANABOLIC STEROIDS AND TESTOSTERONE MYTHS

The flow of life depends on complex organisms composed of chemicals, enzymes and molecules, bound up in teeny bags called cells, working in harmony to bring us satisfaction and good health. Our hormones are by far the most interesting of these microscopic components of life because of their incredible power, flexibility and uncanny ability to self-regulate while juggling the development of our entire body.

Hormones of the exact composition and strength we need for life hover in our cells at conception and stay with us until our last heartbeat. Our self-repairing and self-regulating system becomes a fundamental part of our physiology and keeps us healthy during times of stress or disease. The ability of our hormones to modify genes and affect future generations is an awesome aspect of the *power of hormones*.

Some men have attempted to harness this power in the quest for the perfect body or the strength of Hercules. Boosting their hormones artificially may not have hurt some body builders, but the search for an easier way to boost their musculature has created new uses and a new language for testosterone—the Big T.

In this chapter I will provide a general overview of the use of anabolic steroids, not only for this generation but also for generations to come. The appeal of lifestyle drugs will increase as the population ages and the Internet gives anyone access to a pharmacy and the ability to self-prescribe.

Anabolic Steroids and the Search for the Perfect Body

If you have a teenage son, whether you know it or not, he may be experimenting with anabolic steroids. Before we find out what goes wrong with such a program of self-administered steroids, let's look at some of the beneficial ways these hormones affect your muscles and physical strength.

The opposite of an anabolic or bodybuilding steroid is a catabolic or destructive one. For example, when we exercise strenuously, tissue breaks down, and medical people call this breakdown of tissue catabolism. Other catabolic states include cancer, malnutrition, AIDS Wasting Syndrome plus muscle wasting conditions such as muscular dystrophy or multiple sclerosis. Anabolic steroids have the ability to block the breakdown of tissue and reverse undesirable weight loss while increasing strength and stamina.

Steroids are testosterone derivatives used to treat a variety of medical conditions, ranging from muscle wasting to severe anemia. Today they are popular for enhancing athletic performance and muscular development. To achieve this purpose, testosterone must be chemically modified to enhance its anabolic, or bodybuilding, effects rather than its androgenic or masculinizing activity. The result is a synthetic, injectable derivative of testosterone that would last for days to weeks.

The resulting anabolic steroid boosts nitrogen levels in any body, promoting protein synthesis, muscle growth and the multiplication of red blood cells. An abundance of nitrogen allows the cells to hang on to extra nitrogen needed to form amino acids, the building blocks of protein. This effect, combined with a greater than the average intake of high-calorie, high-protein foods causes muscle tissue to grow in size. Muscles then enlarge as a result of increased activity.

Surplus hormones can sabotage our self-regulating endocrine system, creating trouble for a man's heart and his blood pressure. Too much testosterone might even cause sudden cardiac death or a heart attack. How? By exercising to excess, increasing the size of the heart muscle, leading to an irregular heart rate and poor health.

While testosterone and its steroid derivatives do promote rapid healing of muscles, ligaments and tendons, they do not exactly make muscles grow. Instead of feeling soreness and aching in their joints and muscles after a workout, bodybuilders using anabolic androgenic steroids have a shorter recovery time. They can return to the gym the next day feeling rejuvenated and ready for more intense exercise. No wonder their muscles get so huge!

The major muscles of our arms, legs and back are the same ones we had when we were 13 years old—they are just bigger. Bodybuilders may measure their muscle power in pounds, but strength comes from muscles, tendons and ligaments, not mass. The anabolic (bodybuilding) effect of testosterone on the androgen receptors is a bonus for men and a curse for women.

The strengthening effect of testosterone supplements can help older men with hypogonadism overcome muscle weakness. By following a carefully managed program, these men can enjoy testosterone's anabolic effects and watch their muscles grow in size and strength. Sounds easy! This may tempt you to treat yourself with steroids. Don't go there. Don't listen to your gym buddy or be taken in by false advertising. The stakes are too high. The super-high doses of testosterone can convert to estrogen, feminizing men.

Have you ever wondered why women don't build big muscles when they exercise? The main reason is that they have much lower

233

testosterone levels—approximately one tenth those of men. Women can firm and tone their muscles by lifting weights and their lean body mass will increase slightly. But, if they use anabolic steroids, they will develop muscles just like men. Yes, women can bulk up too. But it doesn't just end there.

Women using powerful anabolic steroids may feel good about increasing their muscle mass, but it startles the rest of us when we notice hair growing on their faces and chest. Their breasts shrink and they develop a deep, masculine voice. These are the masculinizing (androgenic) effects of testosterone and they are *not* reversible.

An average teenage girl naturally produces somewhere around one half milligram (0.5 mg) of testosterone a day. At one time East German sports authorities routinely prescribed steroids to young adolescent girls in doses of up to 35 milligrams a day-*seventy times* the normal amount. After the fall of the Berlin Wall, an investigation into former female athletes found that most retained masculinized physiques and voices, years after discontinuing their steroid therapy.

Other side effects were far more serious. Women came forward with tales of deformed babies, inexplicable tumors, liver dysfunction, internal bleeding and depression, but only after *stopping* their steroids. It was as if their systems suddenly went haywire. The same thing happens to men after ending steroid use. I often get letters from young men who are experimenting with self-injection of anabolic steroids. Here's a typical one.

A young patient I'll call Sean told me that he had taken blood tests and had managed to buy injectable testosterone in Mexico. Sean read the numbers wrong and assumed the concentration was half what it was. As a result he gave himself a double dose. After self-injecting 600 milligrams of the product, Sean saw his test measurements jump sky high. A normal reading of DHT (dihydrotestosterone) for an adult male is 30 to 85ng/dl.

Sean's level 36 hours after the injection was 5,023 ng/dl; both his free testosterone and total testosterone levels were off the charts. Sean was concerned about the effect of this super dose on his testicles and liver, as he should have been. Then again, he should have been more concerned about becoming addicted to these high levels of testosterone, an ever-increasing problem for users of injectable steroids.

Evidence has surfaced showing that testosterone or hormones such as oxytocin can generate beta-endorphins, which play a role in the brain's addiction potential. These chemicals can alter the perception of both pain and pleasure. Normally only opioid substances can affect these receptors, but anabolic steroids can mimic some of their opioid-like action. Feelings of power and euphoria induced by super high levels of steroids may also contribute to addiction.

The sport of bodybuilding abounds with statistics and stories of premature deaths from steroid abuse. Most are hushed up while competitors continue to buy their steroids illegally and self-medicate. Nonetheless, bodybuilders are not criminals and should not be prosecuted for trying to improve themselves by using steroids. John Hoberman points out the social and ethical implications of testosterone use in *Testosterone Dreams,* stating that enhancement medicine is an accepted part of our culture and professional sports. Major league baseball and the Olympics both give testimony to hormone doping. Recently, more stringent laws have been passed but in the past, a slap on the wrist was the only penalty.

Sean, the part-time bodybuilder, eventually confessed his overuse of prescribed testosterone and explained it to me like this. "It's amazing how huge you can look with the right lighting, a good tan and a clean shave. Bodybuilders like to show off their bodies and feel pride in the work they do to develop musculature to the max. Roids help us get bigger muscles. An athlete on the juice can recover fast enough to work a different body part every day".

"Many of these men wouldn't need to resort to such boosting measures if more doctors would be willing to diagnose and treat men who feel they cannot develop sufficient muscle mass, regardless of expending tremendous efforts." He continued, "By the way, I meant to ask you, do your patients stay on your testosterone cream year round? (Yes) Do they cycle it? (No) Do they need any kind of drug to restart their own testosterone production? (They were hypogonadal to begin with)."

"You must have been thrilled to see the recent press coverage on testosterone supplementation. I would not be surprised if steroids were taken off the Schedule 3 list in a couple of years. I would hope that if the pubic gets interested in testosterone supplementation and people want it, lawmakers would reconsider and accept the wonderful benefits of testosterone supplementation in appropriate dosages. What do you think?"

My answer to Sean is that anabolic steroids have both good and bad effects, but they will never be taken off the controlled substance list. Physicians are medically trained to monitor hormone use; self-medicating addicts are not! Some men feel a need for steroids or more steroids even if they're already taking them, just to grow bigger after they have reached their goals. Remember, anabolic hormones only increase protein metabolism and speed healing.

Neither testosterone nor DHT supplements can give anyone a muscular body unless they workout hard. Only the regular effort involved in weight-bearing exercises can make muscle tissue and its supporting structure, collagen, grow in response to the stimulated protein metabolism. Testosterone simply makes it less painful to gain more muscle mass. Recovery time can be cut in half with testosterone.

Most men fail to understand that they are merely increasing muscle size and not the number of muscle cells when they utilize anabolic steroids. They also ignore the possibility of severe side effects from excessive use of steroids: hypertension, acne, hardening of the arteries, increased blood clotting, jaundice, liver cancer, tendon damage, loss of fertility and psychological problems. Additional complications for men include reduced fertility, shrinkage of sex organs and breast enlargement or gynecomastia. Women taking steroids can develop irreversible masculine characteristics such as deep voices.

Many athletes lift far more weight than is necessary to develop a muscular physique. Muscles grow in response to the presence of adequate testosterone or the more anabolic form called DHT. A complex interaction of diet, hormones and exercise plus the anabolic effects of testosterone helps muscles grow. At the risk of repeating myself, let me emphasize that hormones, especially androgenic anabolic steroids (AAS), affect many organ systems and should not be used without medical supervision. There is a place in medicine for these powerful hormones but they should not be mixed with other drugs or alcohol.

Alcohol is well known for its sedative effect or the way it relieves people of their inhibitions. Anabolic steroids block this effect and alter behavior by increasing the pleasure they feel from dopamine-dominant behavior. All at once, alcohol opposes the sedative effects of serotonin. What this means is that men using steroids can enhance their ability to "hold their liquor," giving them the feeling they are neither tired nor drunk, so they imagine they can drive safely while under the influence. Sadly they often end up as roadway fatalities.

Hormones such as testosterone directly affect physical characteristics in powerful ways. Professional athletes, men who are active in gyms and the average Joe should have access to testing to see if their testosterone levels are adequate for normal functioning. A physician should administer all restorative efforts in order to avoid some of the common problems of overdosing such as abscesses, severe acne, swollen breast tissue and small testicles.

Hoberman says it won't be that easy. An estimated five million individuals in the United States are current or past users of anabolic steroids. In the U.S. alone 50 percent of anabolic steroid users self-administer their hormones by an injection into their muscle tissue. About 25 percent of adolescent steroid abusers, including high school girls, share needles, placing them at risk for sharing HIV and hepatitis infections as well.

We have seen that hormones are affected by light, growing old and imbalances in the way your neurotransmitters work. We have discussed feedback systems that your hormones use to regulate the activities of other hormones circulating in your bloodstream. What happens if you overdose on these wonderful hormones? Embracing the "more is better" concept, some athletes experiment on themselves without supervision or any sort of monitoring. These guys are determined to possess a perfectly developed body, but too often their dreams turn into nightmares.

You cannot affect one system without affecting another—there is a true balance in your body and you have to respect it. You can always find a qualified physician who will carefully monitor any supplementation program you undertake.

Testosterone: The Misunderstood Hormone

We have always assumed that testosterone enabled the brain to tolerate risk and peril and that testosterone levels were closely related to the pursuit of risky objectives and aggression. Our primitive forefathers leading the dangerous hunt were most likely dominant males with the highest testosterone.

Our current definition of danger has escalated beyond chasing caribou or fighting wild sabertooth tigers, to include binge drinking, drunk driving and unprotected sex. These forms of risk do not need a boost from testosterone. It is incorrect to assume that high levels of testosterone motivate today's unsafe behavior in the same way that they did during the cavemen time.

Make no mistake. Testosterone is still the most important male hormone in charge of the development of male sexuality and manliness. Men with higher testosterone levels are often successful and very motivated while those with low testosterone levels are far more likely to be moody and insecure. To compensate for their low self-esteem, some men with low testosterone seem to look to physical and emotional thrills to stimulate them. They seek out dangerous behaviors such as drug misuse, sex with multiple partners or skydiving. Many of these low-T men have higher than normal levels of both estrogen and cortisol.

In our society today, the "common wisdom" is that binge drinking, drunk driving and risky sex result from high levels of testosterone. This is not true. We now have convincing evidence that testosterone is not the primary factor in risky behavior. A research team led by Dr. J. C. Rosenblitt at Florida State University studied college students and found that, contrary to popular belief, a positive relationship between testosterone and sensation-seeking behavior did *not* exist in this population.

The testosterone myth regarding prostate cancer or increased risk of this type of cancer is widespread. As the evidence shows, there is nothing to support a link between elevated testosterone and prostate cancer. In fact the link seems to be stronger between lower testosterone and prostate cancer, at least in families where someone has died from this disease.

Fear of testosterone as an unsafe drug is based on misconceptions about the function of this hormone in your body. Of course we know that testosterone is a powerful enhancement drug and that its abuse can lead to serious disorders. Nevertheless, for men with a testosterone deficiency, medically sound supplementation offers such a broad range of benefits that it cannot possibly be considered "a dangerous drug."

Over the past decade, my patients have used hormone replacement in various forms. Many people have sent me positive letters regarding their experience with transdermal testosterone products. They generally feel happier, calmer, more motivated and as a result they are enjoying life. They tell me that they awaken with erections after years of erectile difficulties. Nowadays they are thriving instead of merely surviving. For a family physician, this is totally gratifying.

As mentioned earlier, the need to survive has influenced our development from the time that men first evolved as hunters. Dangerous, sensation-seeking behavior was essential on a daily basis to bring in game from the hunt. Testosterone enabled the brain to tolerate risk and peril. Caveman leaders and chieftains probably had the highest testosterone levels of their tribes, but this allowed them to lead the group, find wild game and impregnate the most females.

Nearly everybody is born with a perfectly balanced supply of hormones performing their job flawlessly but few of us will maintain that ideal state throughout our lifetimes. Any time we come up short in the hormone department, we experience a less-than-ideal life whether it's in the area of aging, libido, raw physical strength or mental capacity. Hormone supplementation makes a huge difference in the lives of both sexes, restoring self-confidence and optimizing sexual function. Learning about your hormones and how they affect your muscular development or your arousal mechanism will help you find what you need to restore love and passion to your relationship.

Love, Libido and Hormones

Two special neurohormones regulate certain behaviors, including sexuality, intercourse and reproduction. The hormones oxytocin and vasopressin, from the hypothalamus are intimately involved in the sex act but they are light sensitive. In other words, these hormones respond to the amount of available light, which varies with the seasons. Increasing light intensity is the first step in restoring oxytocin and vasopressin levels. A Canadian company, Northern Lights, has developed a high quality and affordable portable light source, SADelite™. I recommend it for my patients suffering from seasonal affective disorder.

Neurohormones can be tapped therapeutically for treating difficulties in human sexuality. Having postulated that oxytocin might be the elusive "love feeling," it was time to test this theory with a few patient volunteers. I conducted a small study to determine if "loving feelings" might be related to oxytocin stimulation in the brain. The supposition—"Is there a hormonal component to falling in love?"

Since we weren't treating any illness, we soon learned that finding lovesick volunteers for the study was impossible since, by definition, people who are in love do not want treatment. As the poet Samuel Daniel stated, *"Love is a sickness full of woes, all remedies refusing."* Therefore we told the men who participated in the trial that the purpose of the study was to measure their volume of ejaculate before and after oxytocin treatment.

The scientific literature indicated that there would be an increase of ejaculate with oxytocin and we wanted to see if this was true. Side effects were mild, if any, so we all felt that it was worth a try. Informed consent was first obtained from all the volunteers.

Then again the true premise we were testing was that love is purely intense affection after an orgasm. In other words, we were verifying the theory that love is a direct emotional response resulting from sexual intercourse (ejaculation and orgasm) that makes two people feel closer. The underlying question was, "Does a man's orgasm create the bond he feels with his mate, or is it oxytocin that increases the loving feelings?" Can we influence these feelings using exogenous hormones?

We tested this assumption in my patients using a diluted oxytocin formula delivered by nasal spray. The sprayer deposited the hormone directly at the base of the "olfactory" brain (via the nasal mucous membranes); from there it diffused to the hypothalamus. You may recall that this region also contains our biologic clock and the sexually dimorphic nucleus.

Each of the men who volunteered was using a transdermal testosterone for at least six months prior to the study to assure that his testosterone deficiency was not a factor. Each couple had complained of the loss of the spark they used to feel when making love. No placebo drug was used. The men all believed that oxytocin served largely as a stimulant for increasing their volume of ejaculate. When used prior to sexual contact, the oxytocin spray elicited these reports from the men:

Steve, my patient who had problems with his depression in the past, said that oxytocin affected the emotional aspect of sex with his wife. "I did not notice the orgasm as stronger physically, but it was definitely stronger emotionally," he said. Steve felt that oxytocin was rather like the emotional counterpart of testosterone. "I felt my wife had a prettier face when I had sex after using the oxytocin. I also felt the act of sex was a bit more sacred." Steve and his wife, Melanie are much happier together as a consequence of this experiment. They have been married for about six years.

Another trial volunteer had a similar experience. Mark, the physician with whom we've had thought provoking discussions, said, "Man, that OXY stuff is fantastic! I will try to describe my response. All I can say is Wow! I felt like a young man again. The amount of sperm just kept on coming. The orgasm, if that's what you call an orgasm, lasted twice as long as it usually does, but the amount of ejaculate was incredible! My partner and I both felt we experienced the best sex ever and fell asleep in each other's arms. When we awoke, we made love again. This is the best marriage enhancer we've experienced in twenty years."

These responses are not surprising, because oxytocin has been found to facilitate bonding in all human beings and it's also intimately involved in sexual relations between couples. Oxytocin becomes more intense when a woman nurses or has an orgasm; it also increases when families travel together or groups of women gather. Oxytocin acts on the uterus, testes, heart, thymus, kidney and pancreas, ever increasing in response to a variety of stimuli such as sucking, birthing and ejaculation.

John, the fireman with the thyroid deficiency, had a different response to oxytocin. "I've already used the oxytocin 12 times," he wrote. "It looks like there's quite a bit left in the bottle, more than the 15 total doses you said were in each bottle. The results have been mixed. Sometimes I ejaculate the same amount, you called the 'baseline,' sometimes twice as much and sometimes three times as much! Very cool, man."

He went on, "Linda was really accommodating with the whole

thing. I'm sure there are other factors at work, like how excited I am at the time of ejaculation and how long a period of foreplay precedes the orgasm. But we had a great night on our 15th anniversary! She looked incredible! I fell in love with her all over again. My orgasms were noticeably more intense, which is great. We're going to try for another pregnancy (seriously this time), as soon as I finish this oxytocin experiment." Linda and John already have five children.

This limited survey demonstrates that while chemical brain mediators and other unknown factors might induce the dazzling "feelings of love," oxytocin somehow plays a part in this complex process. In our uncontrolled study the use of oxytocin as a nasal spray *doubled the volume of ejaculate* for all the men, every one of whom also reported an improvement in their orgasms.

Of course, a few anecdotal cases do not make for breakthrough science and their over-interpretation should be resisted. Scientists prefer to rely on double-blind studies, where neither the patient nor the researcher knows who is using the effective drug, for verifiable evidence of a drug's effectiveness. This was only a preliminary analysis.

A few promising research papers involving oxytocin have already been conducted. Early in the 1970s reports began to appear showing that mating increases blood oxytocin concentrations in animals and humans. A compound that blocks the action of oxytocin seemed to reduce sexual responsiveness in rats after they were given estrogen and progesterone, two hormones that usually promote responsiveness. Similar but less convincing studies found male rats displaying more mounting behavior when oxytocin was delivered to their hypothalamus from an implantable pump.

Results of other animal studies suggest that oxytocin promotes bonding and directs female nursing and birthing behaviors in many species. My personal belief is that the role of oxytocin as a sex hormone and a key player in the behavior we call "couple bonding" will become more evident as research in sexual dysfunction advances. Over time, sexual dysfunction may be shown to be the direct result of a hormonal deficiency. To me, it's not a big reach to believe that hormones are responsible for some of the *emotional* components of making love.

Bonding supplies the behavior humans need to be successful moms and dads for their children and oxytocin stimulates the mechanisms that help us adapt to these parental roles. Here's how oxytocin works. Apparently oxytocin unleashes a chemical that signals endorphins and dopamine receptors in the hypothalamus. Responding to the oxytocin, the brain translates this secret code, promoting a loving, bonding relationship among sexual partners by lowering stress and increasing feelings of closeness. Oxytocin causes couples to feel mellow and focused on making love.

More doctors are taking advanced courses and studying new developments in the field of sexual medicine to learn how to help people with sexual problems. A new medical specialty, Men's Health, has emerged from this interest in male hormones. Men's needs are finally being considered in the same way as women's wishes.

Meanwhile, there are signs that the age of the medical manipulation of human sexuality in all its aspects has already begun. Erection enhancers are coming down the pipelines in a cream form and miraculous drugs to stimulate brain arousal through nasal inhalation are only the beginning. Oxytocin is implicated in the production of sperm and in the ejaculation response. Oxytocin can reverse the delay in ejaculation caused by certain antidepressants and may have a potential role in patients who have sexual side effects from the use of SRIs like Prozac, Zoloft and Paxil.

In the next section we will discuss melanocyte stimulating hormone or alpha-MSH, a hormone that scientists now believe plays a key role in preparing us physically, emotionally and mentally for the sex act—a true brain arousal hormone.

Arousal—The Trigger for Passion in Your Love Life

In her book *Why We Love,* Helen Fisher expresses her belief that passion is a human drive as fundamental as hunger for food. Using Magnetic Resonance Imaging (MRI) she recorded brain activity of people *in love.* She concluded that romantic love is, "deeply embedded in the architecture and chemistry of the human brain." She believes that knowing more about how the brain functions can help us understand divorce, stalking behavior and possibly criminal behavior.

Too many couples complain, "The passion has left our lives." For some that may be true, but it does not have to stay that way. Could hormones provide the "passion activator" that couples need after years of familiarity? Passion can be defined as "intense or overpowering emotion; ardent affection for one of the opposite sex or love." Passion is an essential element of all sexual relationships. Passion is present where there is enthusiasm, love, or desire and in the opposite sense disappears when there is anger, jealousy, or violence.

In a good sense emotionally positive passion provides the essence of sexual responsiveness, including arousal, pleasure and orgasm. Unfortunately, passion sometimes converts to a negative emotion, "a fit of intense and furious anger; rage; a strong impulse tending to physical indulgence; the endurance of some painful infliction; suffering."

Negative passion is associated with the destruction of relationships and the loss of life. Most homicides are committed under the influence of passion gone astray. In spite of that fact, without passion, people feel as if an important facet of their life has been lost. For millions of people the loss of passion or loss of love is blamed on various life stressors, when the true culprit is possibly a hormonal imbalance.

Several hormones and brain chemicals play an essential role in the interconnected feelings of sex, love and passion. Most of these biological compounds are themselves interrelated. We have already discussed oxytocin and testosterone. The melanocortins are a newly discovered group of sex hormones. This tiny army of small protein hormones regulates the release of the hormone cortisol from your adrenals among other activities.

The half dozen or so hormones in the melanocortin system play a key role in regulating our appetite and body weight plus a variety of human conditions such as the color of our skin, how readily we digest fat, how much food we eat, our body's temperature, how our body responds to an inflammation and our memory. One of these regulating hormones, the alpha-melanocyte stimulating hormone or *a*-MSH, elicits physical responses such as grooming, stretching and yawning as well as penile erection. Quite an interesting collection of behaviors!

We have seen that androgens and oxytocin work together in human sexuality and doctors may one day prescribe oxytocin for persons with orgasm or ejaculation difficulties or couples who have bonding issues. The rapidly increasing number of sex clinics will play the major role in delivering these new therapies. Sexual arousal, orgasm and passion can return to your life with the restoration of proper hormonal balance or maybe the use of *a*-MSH. From my perspective, love and sex are complimentary and essential for normal intimacy. Still, positive passion is indispensable for the enjoyment of life!

9

THE FUTURE IS NOW...

Fully informed women can directly benefit their male partners and of course, themselves by understanding how hormones influence their intertwined lives. Small decisions have important consequence for your welfare and that of your mate and children. Finding ways to offset the plunge in your partner's hormones over time will benefit you. You can help your loved ones reach the goal of clean living. Why is this so important?

There are five valuable messages about hormones that I want to leave with you. These five declarations encompass what it takes to keep your hormones in balance so that you can both enjoy life and sex to the max.

Before we get started, please consult with your doctor. Hormone requirements vary greatly at different ages and from individual to individual. Share the information in this book with your physician and hopefully with his guidance you will reach new heights of happiness.

1. The "sexy trio" renews youthfulness—use it, as you need it.

In reading this book, you have come to understand that hormones play a major role in sexual function; for example, progesterone, oxytocin, vasopressin and *a*-MSH are intimately involved in many aspects of arousal. The "sexy trio"—testosterone, progesterone and estrogen work together to assure vigorous sexual performance. In addition to a heightened sexual drive, men with well-adjusted hormones have a leaner, younger-looking body, stronger muscles and tougher bones. As do women! Testosterone promotes healthy hearts by delaying hardening of the arteries and weakening of the heart muscle. Elderly people with higher levels of free testosterone have improved memories and less age-related senility.

Estrogen therapy once promised "eternal youth" to women, only to fail miserably to live up to its promise. Still we shouldn't overlook estrogen's positive effects on your skin, hair, bones and brain. Estrogen is known to cause cancer when used exogenously (source from outside your body) but it also increases blood flow in the brain in addition to preventing some of the degenerative changes that occur in dementia.

Move over estrogen. Make way for testosterone, the hormone that can take credit for helping women live longer than men. Yes, as women age, their testosterone levels go up while men's levels go down. This effect may decrease a woman's risk of heart disease and dementia and delay some of the effects of aging, particularly on her muscles and her bones.

Slowing down the speed of aging has been a goal of modern medicine since its inception. As we roll through the first years of the new millennium, slowing down the rate at which we grow old is high on the wish list of baby boomers, including doctors, who are now looking at their retirement years. Thousands of companies offer hundreds of pills, creams or powders and dozens of regimens promising to block the ravages of time.

Though it has not been proven yet, it is possible for you to *look younger* if your hormones are maintained at "youthful" levels. The question turns out to be, is that what Mother Nature intended? Achieving an optimal hormonal balance does not simply happen by taking more hormones. You should be aware that other factors, such as genetics, diet and exercise play key roles in fine-tuning your hormone system, whether you are male or female.

The genetic influences are only part of the picture. Your hormones are controlled on a day-to-day basis by the action of your hypothalamus and pituitary. Your nervous system continually modifies the transport of these hormones, responding to changes in your internal environment through the ordinary processes of growth, maturity and aging. Some of us do improve with age, like fine wines, while others, regardless of their hormone level, simply decline; but in everybody, getting older is undeniably unavoidable.

Testosterone replacement therapy (TRT) delivered through the skin delays osteoporosis and senility and prevents the loss of motivation we all inevitably experience. The accumulation of excess abdominal fat that contributes to adult onset diabetes shrinks with testosterone stimulation. Testosterone improves insulin sensitivity, sexual function and even depression.

These treatments are not without some risk. Various factors including estradiol or E2 have been implicated in sex organ-related cancers. Estrogen can make tumors grow by increasing their blood supply and dihydrotestosterone or DHT in the presence of high estrogen may be a major trigger for prostate cancer. Testosterone is ultimately the source of all DHT and E2.

This is where progesterone comes in. Progesterone can block both the conversion of testosterone to E2 and/or its metabolism to DHT. Progesterone is interchangeable with testosterone, performing as a neurosteroid in the brain. It can either act as a tranquilizer or improve a man's snoring and breathing.

Binding proteins like SHBG amplify hormone regulators in the brain. Research by Jack Caldwell at the University of Illinois, proved that SHBG acts like a switch, turning sex hormones off and on. The "sexy trio" may intensify sexual arousability receptors, but it's SHBG that pushes the button. Prior to Caldwell's research, we believed that hormones bound to SHBG were *ineffective*. It was concluded that only free or bioavailable hormones could exert beneficial effects in the body. It's far more complicated than that.

At this point in time, physicians need to do more than merely identify hormone deficiencies. We need to measure SHBG and bio-available hormones to determine the amount of active hormone readily accessible to your body. Researchers continue to investigate the unique role your hormone distribution system plays in determining the ultimate availability of a hormone to its specific receptor. In other words, why these hormones work so uniquely in different individuals, depends on you.

2. You don't have to wait for your doctor to diagnose hypogonad-ism—check your hormone level before it's too late.

The only way to determine your ideal hormonal reading is to test it when you are younger. Good news! You don't have to wait for a doctor to test you or your partner. You can verify hormone levels by sending a saliva sample for screening to a reliable lab.

To start with, take steps to assure that your loved one does not suffer from hypogonadism. Begin by having your lover ask his doctor to measure his free testosterone levels. If the results are lower than they should be or if sexual problems such as lack of libido or inability to orgasm exist, ask the medical practitioner to correct any deficiencies. Much of the sexual dysfunction humans experience is related to low testosterone levels and lack of exercise. A regular high-intensity exercise program and an active sex life have been proven to keep hormones at optimal levels for healthy aging.

More than 70 million people have unsatisfactory sex lives. Thirteen million men in the US suffer from hypogonadism, or extremely low levels of testosterone. The numbers for women are undoubtedly higher because when a woman's ovaries are removed by a total hysterectomy, this automatically induces a lack of testosterone.

Although heavy exercise can boost testosterone levels, those men spending a lot of time working out in the gym to improve their physical performance may not be pushing those levels high enough. If your significant other is healthy but has a testosterone deficiency, it is far easier to restore normal levels with a testosterone supplement than by spending hours at a sports center.

For the most part, too many doctors are blind to the benefits of testosterone therapy. This can be a critical mistake for men and women whose sex life, mental health and general fitness are woefully lacking as a result of hypogonadism. Some family physicians look the other way and try to pacify their patients with vague assurances that they're "normal." Others might go too far in the opposite direction and prescribe testosterone for conditions other than hypogonadism.

Your man should learn to listen to the messages testosterone and its active products are sending through his body. He will have to take medically advised steps to correct any sexual dysfunction because he may not have enough sex hormones in his system. Have your spouse ask a doctor to test his hormone levels; you may both be surprised at the results. Prevention is still the best tactic.

3. Toxic chemicals lead to the chronic diseases of aging

Almost daily we hear about another way our world has become contaminated with pollution. Chemical poisons are continually released into our environment from industrial wastes, auto fumes, landfill breakdowns and drugs we flush down the toilet. Ironically, as we bring better medical products to the marketplace, we suffer from the by-products of this innovation as many of these end up in our sewers and waterways.

Polluting chemicals interfere with the function of your endocrine system and for this reason they are named *endocrine disruptive chemicals* or EDCs. Evidence from ongoing research passes the blame for many chronic diseases, weakened immune systems and the premature decline in testosterone onto these EDCs. One alarming effect caused by the onslaught of estrogen from the environment is the tilt of the ratio of testosterone to estrogen in favor of *estrogen excess*. Too much estrogen is bad for both men and women. A surplus of estrogen not only creates a lowered sex drive but also an increased risk of a wide variety of sex-organ-related cancers.

Pollution is the price we pay for human progress. Nonetheless, we should all support policies at the local, regional and national level for a reasonable use of our country's resources. We must appeal to our government to focus on clean air and water rather than subsidizing beef and dairy production and the tobacco, oil and coal industries. We need to clean up our own backyards instead of waiting for some government action.

As a nation we must stop the contamination of our rivers and streams with drug-laden animal manures, environmental estrogens and toxic wastes. Our environment is too precious to waste on breeding organisms that are resistant to antibiotics and multiplying polluting chemicals that can destroy our future, our fertility—and inevitably our health.

Follow a plant-based (vegan) diet by avoiding meat and animal products. You will improve your health! Vegans have even less heart disease, diabetes and arthritis than vegetarians and less cancer than omnivores. Choosing from the abundance of complex carbohydrate and non-meat foods that provide high quality protein will help you maintain your weight. Garden organically—grow salad greens, herbs and other vegetables in your own garden! It's fun and inexpensive.

Don't hesitate to demand accountability from your local elected representatives for the quality of your food and water supply.

4. Ask your doctor for bioidentical hormones in place of synthetics.
"When something is "bioidentical," it is structurally identical to the substance as it physically occurs in your body. Most bioidentical estrogens and progesterone come from soy (estrogen) or yams (progesterone). The hormones are extracted from the plant source, processed to be similar to the hormones in a woman's body." (Hormone Therapy Options: Bioidentical Hormones—follows in the Appendix A (For Women Only).

For decades, injections of testosterone have been the standard for delivering testosterone. Injectable testosterone products are synthetic, functional and relatively inexpensive. A major drawback to injecting testosterone was that blood level of hormone rose rapidly after the shot and then dropped almost as rapidly. The wildly fluctuating amounts of testosterone result in mood disorders and withdrawal symptoms. Many doctors try to get around this problem by injecting weekly instead of monthly in an attempt to stop the roller-coaster effect of an injection. This only creates another set of problems.

Thanks to molecular biology and pharmaceutical engineering, it is now possible to create a "micelle" of testosterone, which will penetrate *intact* skin without damage or drying the skin. The testosterone molecule sits within the micelle, which transports it between cells. These "intelligent gels" can change properties at body temperature and safely deliver hormones into the bloodstream.

The most effective delivery for hormones is through the skin, a method known as *transdermal* delivery. One system uses large plastic patches, which contain a reservoir of hormone suspended in alcohol and a membrane that controls its release. The suspension is similar to the alcohol-based gels, which are just as effective as testosterone shots but safer and more expensive.

Unfortunately, testosterone patches and gels can be irritating to the skin and require quite a bit of material to reach a therapeutic dose in men. High potency gels are not considered safe for approval because the FDA established guidelines to regulate the amount of testosterone in a preparation to limit its abuse. This restriction has created an expensive option for those men who don't want to jab hormones suspended in oil into their buttocks. Fortunately, a new"higher potency, 10-percent testosterone cream has been formulated to eliminate this problem and it is currently available from a few compounding pharmacists in the United States.

Many techniques have been promoted to keep you from growing old, but no proven therapies turn back the hands of time, without unwanted side effects, even on a temporary basis. We will all age in spite of future medical miracles, but by restoring your hormones to more youthful levels through treatment with bioidentical hormones (BHRT), you can help your husband or your mate live in good health. I must caution you that we haven't yet discovered all the secrets about our hormones and how to optimize them for the healthiest results.

5. What Can You Do To Stay Healthy?

The secret to living in harmony with all your hormones is "balance." If your mate's hormone levels are below normal and he experiences lackluster sexual performance, ask him to discuss his concerns with his doctor. He might benefit from bringing those subnormal levels into equilibrium.

Health is a state of body and mind. Good health is the surest way to slow down aging. We have all heard about the importance of diet and exercise, why don't we listen? Diets high in grains, fruits and vegetables contain all the essential vitamins and minerals one needs to stay healthy. Zinc, selenium and the Vitamin E complex of tocopherols may even block the conversion of testosterone to estrogen and help to control SHBG levels.

Phytochemicals are found in seeds, nuts, red clover and avocados, which also provide essential fatty acids similar to those in fish oils. Such compounds, especially Vitamin D, not only help maintain prostate health but also help tilt the ratio in favor of the most favorable estrogen and free testosterone levels.

Traditional American diets that are high in protein and fat play a role in elevating SHBG (sex hormone binding globulin). SHBG reduces the amount of obtainable sex hormones and regulates their availability in your brain. Your favorite American foods, especially those you buy at fast food restaurants or in the prepared food section of the supermarket, contain high fat loaded with environmental compounds. These chemicals exert estrogen-like effects increasing SHBG and blocking the action of testosterone. Without doubt, these foods contribute to heart disease, diabetes, obesity and cancer.

You can make known the dangers of hormones found in your

food and the environment to your friends and neighbors. Sorry to say, a balanced diet alone is not enough to maintain high levels of hormones forever. Certainly, the relative amounts of SHBG-bound testosterone increase making less testosterone available to the androgen receptor. When a man or woman's bioavailable testosterone falls below normal, the appropriate testosterone supplement can reverse many of the devastating effects of deficiency. Balanced hormones are essential for a vibrant life and healthy aging.

Do not make any changes in prescription drugs until you see your own doctor.

Now It's Up To You

Our hormones talk to us whether we are awake or asleep. They endow the human body with an internal language and control our cycles, our brain function and our emotions. They send us signals 24 hours a day, seven days a week, working for us efficiently and continuously. They give us up-to-date information about any declining levels or hormonal imbalances, but we must pay attention to them.

Modern medicine offers practical solutions to many hormone-related problems. The man you love does not have to put up with many of the problems generally accepted as a part of growing old. In short, it's time to stop complaining about how bad he feels and do something about it. His journey towards optimal health may be long and sometimes confusing, but it is always worthwhile. Before you can help your spouse with his hormones, you need to know how they work in the male body. As a woman you can benefit from this book's suggestions but you must pass this information on to your loved one.

As soon as the man in your life mentions that he is too tired to have sex, you know there is a problem. When he goes on to say he is worried about keeping his erection or feels he can no longer satisfy you, it's time to make an appointment with his doctor.

I am going to sum up what we covered.

Any sexual problem is part of a much larger medical condition. In addition to hormone supplements, other factors are involved but the adequacy of hormone levels should be considered first. Remember that most doctors are not endocrinologists and a lot of this information is new to them. Interested physicians can always incorporate the guidelines available from the endocrine society as part of their patients' treatment plan. Men shouldn't blame doctors who don't necessarily have all the latest information about testosterone therapy.

This book helps fill the gap with important new facts about bioidentical hormones and provides access to online, legitimate sources. *A Woman's Guide to Men's Health* represents one approach to your good health, but there are many other therapies besides hormone balancing. Seeing a specialist can certainly help but your doctor should still perform baseline hormone testing.

Physicians should not simply write a prescription for an erection enhancer for any patient complaining of erectile dysfunction. Patients resent being tossed a Viagra or Cialis tablet when they complain about not feeling sexual any longer. *Healthy sex is not simply a matter of erections.*

Living and loving more intensely depend on more than sexual relationships. A well-balanced life implies a genuine concern for others as well as caring for your significant other. Life is more than simply having sex, earning a living or eating and sleeping. We all need to enjoy music, plant a garden and relish precious friendships. More than in the past, our body's hormones are under siege. Hormones hold the secret to the *"joi de vivre"* we all seek.

Quality of life issues are vital. Everyone wants to enjoy his or her life till the end. In addition to diet, exercise and the avoidance of harmful substances, optimal hormone balancing is an important ingredient in reaching this objective. Slowly and cautiously, hormone replacement therapy is becoming the standard of care for both men and women.

Consider the information and the numerous recommendations provided in this book as one doctor's opinion. Not all physicians agree with this view. For those who wish to contact me or consult on any questions that might arise, addresses and website locations are provided. Hopefully this guide has given you some insight into the fascinating world of your hormones and how they affect your body.

You can improve the quality and quantity of your life by benefiting from hormonal therapy now and for many years to come. Aging well and keeping your brain sharp requires more than simply following a good diet and getting your hormones checked regularly. Andrew Weil presents twelve suggestions for healthy aging in his new book, *Healthy Aging*. I highly recommend it. Modern medicine has at its disposal all the tools needed to insure that you live your life free of pain and suffering with enough time to reach your goals and dream your dreams. If you're tired of feeling older than your age, you should recognize the profound effects of hormonal balance on your future health and sex life today!

Appendix A

BIOIDENTICAL HORMONES
(FOR WOMEN ONLY!)

Reproduced by permission from the National Women's Health Resource Center, Inc.

With all the bad news about hormone replacement therapy over the past few years, is it any wonder that more women than ever are now searching for alternatives to treat their menopausal symptoms? As a result, there is increasing interest in ostensible "natural" herbal products and in treatment options known as bioidentical hormones. Unfortunately, there's nearly as much confusion about the meaning of "natural" and "bioidentical" female hormones as there was about hormone therapy in 2002, when the first results of the Women's Health Initiative (WHI) were released. Early results from that study indicated that postmenopausal women using a combination estrogen/progestin medication, Prempro®, faced a slightly increased risk of breast cancer, heart disease, stroke and blood clots. The risks prompted the U.S. Food and Drug Administration (FDA) to mandate warning labels on all estrogen products advising women to use the least amount of hormone necessary for the shortest duration to treat menopausal symptoms.

In the aftermath, millions of women quit their hormone therapy cold turkey—no matter what form they were taking. However, many were surprised by the return of menopausal symptoms they'd thought long gone. Since then, however, newer hormone formulations have been approved, more intensive review of the data has raised some questions about the WHI study itself and, slowly but surely, millions of women are returning to the option of using hormones to treat menopausal symptoms. Now if a woman decides to use hormones, it's more a question of which type of therapy best meets her individual menopausal needs than whether she will use hormone therapy or not. This *Women's Health Update* will help you understand your options when it comes to hormone therapy and separate fact from fiction.

Fact 1: Your body makes three different kinds of estrogen.

These are: estradiol, or E 2, the primary estrogen produced during your reproductive years; estrone, or E 1, the primary estrogen generated during your menopausal years; and estriol, or E 3, the weakest form of estrogen, primarily available during pregnancy when it is created by the placenta. Each form works differently in different parts of your body.

Fact 2: "Natural" is a marketing term, not a medical term.

Just because a medication or supplement is labeled "natural" doesn't mean it's any safer than a drug or supplement created in a laboratory. In fact, there is usually more evidence that a pharmaceutical medication is safer than an over-the-counter product made from soy, or an estrogen created in a compounding pharmacy (a pharmacy that custom-mixes medications). That's because pharmaceutical manufacturers must submit to strict testing to receive FDA approval and close FDA monitoring of all manufacturing to insure purity; closely track distribution to stop counterfeiting; and submit any reports of adverse events relating to their product to the FDA. Manufacturers of supplements and compounded hormones do not have to follow any of these requirements.

Fact 3: Women today can choose from many options to treat their menopausal symptoms.

It is important to understand that the WHI focused on just two forms of hormone therapy- Premarin, a conjugated estrogen made from the urine of pregnant mares and Prempro, which contains Premarin plus a synthetic progestin, a strong form of progesterone labeled medroxyprogesterone acetate, or MPA. While these products have been on the market for many years, there are now many new hormone formulations in varying dosages to consider for symptom relief. These options range from pills to creams to patches to a gel.

Fact 4: As with any medication, all forms of hormone therapy have the potential for side effects.

Whether it was made in a lab or specially created for an individual woman in a compounding pharmacy, all hormones have certain side effects and risks. For instance, estrogen normally present in your body until menopause has been implicated in a woman's risk of breast and uterine cancer, with many studies finding that women with naturally higher levels of two forms of estrogen- estradiol and estrone-have a higher risk of breast cancer than women with lower levels.

Your body is designed to function with lower amounts of circulating estrogen following menopause. Using hormone therapy isn't a requirement; it's an option available to women who need relief from symptoms associated with declining estrogen levels during the menopause transition, such as vaginal dryness, hot flashes and night sweats. Commonly reported side effects of estrogen hormone therapy include: headache, breast pain, irregular vaginal bleeding or spotting, stomach cramps/bloating, nausea and vomiting and hair loss.

Fact 5. If hormone therapy is indicated, the FDA recommends that it should be prescribed at the lowest effective dose for the shortest time needed.
Using this guideline is the safest option for all women who choose to use hormone therapy. Your health care professional will determine the dose and timing depending on your health profile and response to therapy. Finding the dose and formulation that works best to relieve your symptoms may take some time (and perhaps varying doses and hormone therapy options) and should be re-evaluated on a regular basis.

Defining Bioidentical

When something is "bioidentical," it is structurally identical to the substance as it normally occurs in your body. Most bioidentical estrogens and progesterone come from soy (estrogen) or yams (progesterone). Once the hormones are extracted from the plant source, they can be processed and used by a woman's body. There are two main types of bioidentical hormones: those that are FDA-approved and commercially available with a prescription, such as Estrace and EstroGel and those that are mixed on an individual basis for women in compounding pharmacies, which are not FDA-approved. Estrogen products manufactured via compounding are typically labeled "bi-estrogen" or "tri-estrogen," since they contain varying amounts of the two or three types of estrogen. The individual prescription is typically created based on a saliva test that identifies the forms of estrogen in which a woman is deficient. However, saliva testing is not reliable; nor is it used to determine dosage or to monitor therapy.

Safety and Regulation of Bioidentical Hormones

If you choose to have your bioidentical hormones custom-made for you in a compounding pharmacy, you need to understand that their production, the purity of the product and the safety of the dose designed for you are unregulated. Additionally, no safety or efficacy studies (i.e., studies showing how well the drug works) have been conducted or published. While these formulations may use FDA-approved ingredients, the customized formulations are not approved and there are no guidelines for their use. Pharmaceutical bioidentical products, however, are subjected to a rigorous review of their benefits and health risks before they can be marketed. They are only allowed on the market if the benefits outweigh the risks. Additionally, the federal government regulates the quality of pharmaceutical estrogens and progesterone.

Your Hormone Options

Women have numerous FDA-approved options today when it comes to hormone therapy. The following outlines the nine main formulations of FDA-approved hormone therapy available in the United States:

Oral—Most hormone therapy formulations still come in a pill form. The only bioidentical oral form is Estrace (micronized estradiol). (Don't be put off by the word "micronized," it just means that the estrogen particles were made smaller for better absorption.)

Transdermal gel—EstroGel (estradiol gel) is applied once a day to the arm, from wrist to shoulder. This bioidentical estrogen is a clear, odorless gel that dries on the arm in two to five minutes. It doesn't cause the skin to dry out and is approved for the treatment of moderate to severe hot flashes and moderate to severe dryness, itching and burning in and around the vagina.

Lotion—Estrasorb (estradiol topical emulsion) is a bioidentical estrogen. Women apply this white, lotion-like emulsion to both their legs (thighs and calves) on a daily basis. Estrasorb has been approved for treating moderate to severe symptoms of hot flashes and night sweats associated with menopause.

Vaginal cream—Estrogen creams include Estrace (micronized estradiol cream), Ogen (estropipate cream), Ortho dienestrol cream and Premarin (conjugated estrogen cream). These creams are generally used only to treat vaginal symptoms of menopause. Only Estrace is a bioidentical estrogen cream.

Vaginal ring—There are two rings currently available, Femring (estradiol acetate) and Estring (estradiol). Only Estring is a bioidentical form of estrogen in a ring. The ring is a small piece of circular plastic silicone that is inserted into the vagina like a diaphragm, where it releases a steady dose of estrogen for three months, at which point it is replaced. Femring is approved to treat moderate to severe hot flashes, night sweats and vaginal dryness. Estring is approved for the treatment of urogenital complaints related to menopause, including vaginal dryness, urinary urgency (feeling like you suddenly have to go to the bathroom), painful intercourse and painful urination.

Patches—Ranging from smaller than a dime in size to nickel and half-dollar sizes, estrogen patches are typically applied to the abdomen or upper buttock. They are designed to stay on when showering or swimming. They have varied dosing, with some needing to be changed once a week, others twice weekly. However, you have to rotate where you wear the patch and there is a possibility of skin irritation. Bio-identical patches include Vivelle Dot, Alora, Climara, Menostar and Estraderm, which all are estradiol. With the exception of Menostar, which is approved for osteoporosis prevention, these products are approved for a variety of menopause symptoms, including hot flashes and vaginal symptoms.

Vaginal tablet—Less messy than a cream, Vagifem is an estradiol tablet inserted into the vagina via a disposable applicator. The general dose is one tablet daily for the first two weeks, followed by one tablet twice a week. It is bioidentical and generally used only for relief of vaginal symptoms.

Injection—Before there were creams and vaginal pills, there was Delestrogen (estradiol valerate), an injection. Still available in the U.S., this form of estrogen is taken once a month and women are urged to discontinue or taper the dose at three or six month intervals. It is not, however, a bioidentical formulation.

Progesterone—To reduce the risk of endometrial cancer, progesterone is prescribed along with estrogen-only hormone therapy products. There are two forms of bioidentical progesterone currently available: Prometrium (oral capsule) and Prochieve (a vaginal gel).

More information on menopause and hormone therapy is available in the National Women's Health Report, "Menopause: Hormone Therapy &Other Options," available online: http://www.healthywomen.org, or by calling the National Women's Health Resource Center toll-free: 1-877-986-9472.

The Sad Days of Menopause

Men may blame their discomfort on retirement or problems at work, but anyone with constant pain or hot flashes would feel depressed. The hormone problems that cause men to feel depressed fade in comparison with those that women endure. Women become depressed about three times as often as men and are more than twice as likely to suffer bipolar depression with wild mood swings. Scientists believe that women suffer more from depression than men because a larger portion of their brains is devoted to recognizing and processing emotions.

Think about the roller coaster of hormones in a woman's life. She is constantly adjusting to hormone fluctuations. From menstruation and pregnancy to childbirth and menopause, she confronts an array of hormone-driven activities. Some women cannot achieve a perfect balance of all hormones during these real but chaotic phases of life. As a result they may suffer from deficiencies of the key chemicals needed for their brain to function optimally and this can lead to clinical depression.

For example, a woman whose testosterone levels drop while her estrogen levels are rapidly fluctuating is probably going to suffer from some type of depression. This frequently occurs in the condition called post partum depression—becoming depressed soon after giving birth to a baby. With this type of depression the new mother's mood might shift rapidly from elation to despair primarily because of dramatic changes in her hormones. She has now developed a classic case of what is known as post partum psychosis, associated with chaotic mood swings from high to low, an indicator of bipolar depression.

In contrast, women, who are clinically depressed, a condition also known as unipolar depression, are likely to complain of fatigue, distress, increased appetite and excessive sleepiness. Severely depressed women often have trouble getting out of bed in the morning or experience difficulty falling asleep at night. Normally, sexual dreams are an indication of a woman's erotic desire. An "early warning sign" of depression could be fewer dreams of this nature. Women whose testosterone is waning report fewer erotic dreams.

Jan, a young mother, wrote this letter to me, providing a classic example of a person who feels "stressed out" but in actuality has unipolar depression.

"I am 31," she wrote, "and have a highly stressed life." Jan described her situation: three small children, a husband who travels for work, barely any support system and a mom who lives out of town. "I feel worried, anxious and a lot of the time like I am not doing it 'good enough'. I have a hard time getting the appropriate sleep I need and feel miserable and 'mad at the world' in the morning because I didn't sleep as well as I should have."

Sometimes the stress level is better and sometimes worse. "But," she observed, "I do snap out of it and I am OK with the kids and stuff. I just feel overwhelmed a lot and can't get my head straight. I take time-outs quite often for myself, but don't get as many as I should. I wish I could just go with the flow more and handle things better."

I could tell that Jan was worried. I could almost hear her anxious voice when I read her plea, "Can you recommend a mild medication that can help with my anxiousness and my feeling like I want to cry but usually can't even if I tried? I feel I only need something to take the edge off."

Many women like Jan feel distressed most of the time. Their predominant symptom is anxiety, common in both unipolar and bipolar depression. They may be on the edges of clinical depression, but they may think all they need is a tranquilizer-something to "take the edge off." They have no idea that they are seriously depressed. Treating anxiety with calming drugs may work for a short while, but it only masks the problem. If the feelings persist longer than six months, they are probably due to clinical depression, not just stress.

Women who have gone through menopause and feel depressed can cheer up with good news about dehydroepiandrosterone, the DHEA steroid. Experts have determined that menopausal women are deficient in several hormones but when they are treated with DHEA, they may notice improvement in their sense of well-being. Apparently DHEA has a positive effect on the central nervous system. Its primary action seems to be an ordinary increase in estrogen. In addition, post-menopausal women can enjoy higher levels of testosterone following a program of taking DHEA supplements. Higher levels of these male hormones, make women feel better much the same as the effect they have on men. However, men do not seem to respond to DHEA in the same way.

Joyce, a 52-year old interior decorator went through menopause five years before writing to me. "My libido, sexual arousal and responsiveness are now practically non-existent," she wrote. "I wake up every day with hot flashes and pain in my joints. I could probably not do anything sexual even if I wanted to. I love my husband and he loves me. We both miss the closeness of the wonderful physical relationship we once had." Joyce's experience is a classic menopausal reaction and it closely follows the changes that take place in men during the time we call mid-life crisis.

So which is it, Andropause or Menopause that inevitably lowers testosterone? Both are right.... Sooner or later concentrations drop. The following guidelines will let you (whether you are a man or a woman) know where you fall in the "Normal Levels of Testosterone by Age."

Appendix B

NORMAL LEVELS OF TESTOSTERONE BY AGE FOR MALES AND FEMALES

BIOAVAILABLE TESTOSTERONE

Pre-pubertal boys and girls	<0.2 to 1.3 ng/dl
Adult females	1.1 to 14.3 ng/dl
Adult Males	
20 to 39 years	128 to 430 ng/dl
40 to 49 years	3.46 to 17.25 nm or 100 to 497 ng/dl
50 to 59 years	2.77 to 14. 55 nm or 80 to 419 ng/dl
60 to 69 years	2.42 to 12.37 nm or 70 to 356 ng/dl
70 to 79 years	1.45 to 9.62 nm or 64 to 277 ng/dl

TOTAL TESTOSTERONE (SERUM)

Boys

<9.8 years	<3 to 10 ng/dl
9.8 to 14.5 years	18 to 150 ng/dl
10.7 to 15.4 years	100 to 320 ng/dl
11.8 to 16.2 years	200 to 620 ng/dl
12.8 to 17.3 years	350 to 970 ng/dl

Adult males (~prior estimates and *current standards)

~20 to 29 years	10.7 to 28.8 nm or 310 to 830 ng/dl (Schaltz, 2003)
~30 to 39 years	10.4 to 28.8 nm or 300 to 830 ng/dl (Schaltz, 2003)
*40 to 49 years	8.7 to 31.7 nm or 251 to 913 ng/dl
*50 to 59 years	7.5 to 31.4 nm or 216 to 905 ng/dl
*60 to 69 years	6.8 to 29.8 nm or 196 to 859 ng/dl
*70 to 79 years	6.9 to 28.4 nm or 199 to 818 ng/ dl

Adult females

18 to 24 years	0.6 to 2.9 nm or 17 to 84 ng/dl
25 to 34 years	0.30 to2.30 nm or 9 to 66 ng/dl
35 to 44 years	0.10 to 3.20 nm or 3 to 92 ng/dl
45 to 54 years	0.10 to 2.60 nm or 3 to 75 ng/dl
55 to 64 years	0.10 to 2.00 nm or 3 to 58 ng/dl
65 to 75 years	0.10 to 4.00 nm or 3 to 115 ng/dl

FREE TESTOSTERONE (SERUM)

Adult males (~prior estimates and *current standards)

~20 to 50 years	52 to 280 pg/ml (Esoterix Labs)
*40 to 49 years	0.183 to 0.192 nm or 5 to 26 ng/dl
*50 to 59 years	0.146 to 0.770 nm or 4 to 22 ng/dl
*60 to 69 years	0.128 to 0.654 nm or 3.69 to 19 n/dl
*70 to 79 years	0.107 to 0.509 nm or 2.22 to 15 ng/dl

Adult females

18 to 24 years	5.77 to 46.32 pm or 1.66 to 13.36 pg/ml
25 to 34 years	3.02 to 58.24 pm or 0.87 to 16.80 pg/ml
35 to 44 years	1.55 to 47.92 pm or 0.45 to 13.82 pg/ml
45 to 54 years	1.81 to 43.60 pm or 0.52 to 12.57 pg/ml
55 to 64 years	2.03 to 49.28 pm or 0.59 to 14.21 pg/ml
65 to 75 years	1.36 to 52.87 pm or 0.39 to 15.25 pg/m

Normal Levels of Testosterone by Age for Males and Females from two recent studies in men and women.

Testosterone Measurements in Women

Problems of testosterone measurement are further complicated by the fact that the available assays were designed for men, in whom normal testosterone levels range from 300 to 1200 ng/dl, whereas a range of 3 to 115 ng/dl is normal for women. This is a non-specific range and new age-specific levels have been determined for both men and women. (See above).

I have included the values for male hormones from a recent study by Dr. Davis' Women's Health Program at the Department of Medicine at Monash University, Melbourne, Australia. The medical abstract is reproduced below.

ABSTRACT: *"This cross-sectional study of 1423 randomly recruited community based women aged 18 to 75 years, explores the effects of age, natural and surgical menopause on androgen levels in healthy women… We report that serum androgen levels decline steeply in the early reproductive years; do not vary as a consequence of actual menopause and that the postmenopausal ovary appears to be an ongoing site of testosterone production."* (April 2005. Davison et al., androgen levels in adult females: changes with age. Journal of Clinical Endocrinology & Metabolism 2005; 90, (7): 3847-53).

References for new hormone ranges

1. Mohr B, Guay AT, O'Donnell AB, McKinley JB, Morley JE, et al. Normal, bound and nonbound testosterone levels in normally ageing men: results from the Massachusetts Male Ageing Study. Clinical Endocrinology (2005) 62, 64-73

2. Davison SL, R Bell R, Donath S, Montalto JG, Davis SR. Androgen levels in adult females: changes with age. Journal of Clinical Endocrinology & Metabolism. First published April 12, 2005

FDA-approved Laboratories
That Provide Hormone Testing

Esoterix, Inc. (Now with Lab Corp)
4301 Lost Hills Road
Calabasas Hills, CA 91301
www.esoterix.com
800-444-9111

ARUP Labs
500 Chipeta Way
Salt Lake City, Utah 84108
www.arup.com

Nichols Labs (Now With Quest)
1311 Calle Batido
San Clemente, CA 92673
www.nicholsdiag.com

Recommended Laboratory for Salivary Hormone Testing

Diagnos-Techs, Inc.
6620 South 192nd Place, Building
Kent, WA 98032
800-878-3787
diagnos@diagnostechs.com
www.diagnostechs.com

Please visit my website at: www.WellnessMD.com. If you have further questions you can email me at: DRK@wellnessmd.com or www.Kryger.Medem.com for secure and confidential consultations. Online hormone testing can be performed using salivary hormone kits for screening. However, testosterone cannot be prescribed without a medical examination by a physician.

GLOSSARY

A quick survey of this book will reveal that hormones are powerful chemical messengers in the human body, but you may be wondering exactly how they originate, what they do that makes them so powerful and what the words mean. The following glossary should be useful to help you understand the terms and medical jargon used in this book. We highlighted many of the words throughout the book.

5-AR. 5-alpha reductase. An enzyme involved in producing DHT, concentrated in the skin, hair and genital organs and four times higher in balding areas than in the back of the scalp. Without this enzyme it's impossible to become bald or have a sex drive.

ACTH Adrenocorticotropic hormone. A releasing hormone from the pituitary that increases production of adrenal steroids and plays a major role in stress.

ADH. Anti-diuretic hormone. See vasopressin. Stops nighttime urination.

Adrenaline. A chemical transmitter originating in the adrenal gland and causing the "flight or fight" reaction. Also named epinephrine. Used to reverse severe allergic reactions.

Aldosterone. A salt-regulating hormone that comes from the adrenal gland and affects the functioning of the kidney. It interacts with progesterone and affects blood pressure.

Alzheimer's Disease. A degenerative brain disease, which strikes older people and is associated with dementia or loss of memory. Named for a Dr. Alzheimer who first described the disease in his wife but he could not find a cure. The disease seems to have a hereditary component,

Anabolic (bodybuilding) steroids. Synthetic derivatives of testosterone originally developed to treat a variety of medical conditions and used today to enhance athletic performance and muscular development. Also dubbed "roids" or "juice" by the bodybuilding community.

Androderm® Manufactured by Watson Pharmaceuticals. A skin patch delivering testosterone and used for two decades without negative effects other than occasional skin reactions. A similar product is TestoDerm® by Alza Pharmaceuticals. These plastic patches deliver about 5 milligrams of testosterone daily.

AndroGel® Manufactured by Unimed. The first 1% testosterone gel marketed by Solvay pharmaceuticals and approved by the FDA in 2000. Requires one 5-gram packet to deliver about 5 milligrams of testosterone into the blood stream. Now available in a pump delivery system.

Androgens. Male hormones such as testosterone and dihydrotestosterone or DHT. (*andros* means "man" in Greek.) These hormones control sex drive in both men and women.

Andropause. The male equivalent of female menopause. Associated with slow declining hormone levels in men 55 to 70 years of age. Not yet recognized by the American Medical Association.

Androstenedione. A precursor hormone of testosterone. Has potent action in women and can directly convert to the estrogen form-Estrone (E1). Sold for years over-the-counter as food supplement and used by young men to try to increase testosterone but instead increases estrogen. Removed from the market by the FDA in March, 2004. Study from Melbourne, Australia, by Davis and her group provides age-specific levels for women.

Androsterone. The definitive male sex hormone discovered in the testicles in 1931. The first "steroid" hormone known to man.

Anhedonia. People with this problem may stop eating, stop sleeping and develop that flat emotional state, wherein they get no pleasure from anything.

ANS. Autonomic nervous system. Also known as the visceral or automatic system. The ANS transmits impulses from the blood vessels, heart and primary organs to the brain, which simulates mostly automatic or reflex actions such as digestion and childbirth.

Anti-androgen. A substance working in opposition to male hormones and interfering with the action of testosterone. Estrogen and progesterone, for example, are considered are anti- androgens.

Antigens. Substances such as invading viruses or bacteria that are recognized as "foreign" by the immune system, which subsequently produces antibodies to destroy them.

Aromatase. An enzyme complex responsible for the conversion of testosterone to the form of estrogen known as estradiol. Anti-aromatase drugs, such as Tamoxifen, interfere with the formation of estradiol are used in treating breast cancer.

ART. Androgen replacement therapy. A program of male hormone supplementation, effective in treating anemia, wasting diseases such as cancer and AIDS, impotence, hypogonadism, prostrate enlargement and pituitary deficiency. Not yet an accepted therapy for all of the listed conditions.

BGH. Bovine growth hormone. A growth hormone manufactured in cows and used as a supplement to increase the size of cattle. Present in milk and beef but considered "safe for human consumption." There is some evidence that it may be involved in prostate cancer.

BPH. Benign prostatic hyperplasia. Non-cancerous enlargement of the prostate gland, which increases with aging in men and is affected by both estrogen and DHT. Causes men to wake up more than once during the night to urinate and can be treated by 5-AR blockers.

Bulbourethral Reflex. An involuntary reflex of the internal anal sphincter which occurs when the penis is compressed.

Catabolic. Characteristic of tissue breakdown. Catabolic states including cancer, malnutrition, AIDS and multiple sclerosis and are treated with anabolic (bodybuilding) steroids.

Cialis® Manufactured by Lilly/Icos. Tadalafil, a new erection enhancer, marketed to last 36 hours, compared to Viagra, which lasts four to six hours. Dubbed the "weekend pill," Cialis has become a popular sex drug.

Cortical. Related to the cortex, the outer part or "rind" of the brain, including multiple lobes and areas involved in integrating information received from our senses. The cortex or cortical brain controls emotions and holds memories and thought. The cortex is destroyed in Alzheimer's Disease.

Cortisol. A major hormone released by the adrenal glands whenever we feel anxious or stressed or allergic. Regulates our fuel source, blood sugar (glucose) and converts proteins to glucose during times of stress to give us energy to deal with the stressful situation. Too much cortisol can cause confusion and weight gain; too little makes it difficult to handle stress.

Cremasteric Reflex. An involuntary reflex of the muscles in the scrotal sac, which contract when the inner aspect of the thigh is stroked. This reflex is usually present in all males regardless of age.

CRH and CRF. Cortisol releasing hormone or Corticotropin Releasing Factor. A hormone that is released from the pituitary to regulate the production of cortisol by the adrenal glands. CRH blockers are being studied as future antidepressants.

Daidzein. An isoflavone found mostly in soybeans, legumes (red clover) and peas. Daidzein has been shown to have a beneficial effect on some types of cancer and bone health. Daidzein inhibited prostate cancer cell growth without causing DNA damage and may also protect against breast cancer.

DDT. Dichlorodiphenyltrichloroethylene. An insecticide (bug killer) that is highly toxic to both animals and humans. The most widely used insecticide until it was banned in the US in 1972. Still used in Mexico and South America plus in Africa.

DEA. Drug Enforcement Agency. The policing arm of the Federal Drug Administration, involved in preventing abuse and illegal marketing of drugs in the US.

Depo-testosterone or Testosterone enanthate. A long-acting synthetic testosterone injected once every two weeks in men who are testosterone deficient. Often diverted to black market and sold in gyms as "juice."

DES. Diethylstilbestrol. The first synthetic estrogen developed for treating animals. When prescribed for pregnant women, DES created estrogen levels hundreds to thousands of times more potent than estrogen produced normally by the body. As a result babies were born with severe deformities and ambiguous sexual preference.

DHEA. Dehydroepiandrosterone. The primary steroid secreted from the adrenal gland. The DHEA steroid has a positive effect on the central nervous system and is being investigated as a future medication for treating, depression, obesity, heart disease and immune deficiency. Recent Mayo Clinic study stated it had no effect on aging or sex drive.

DHT. Dihydrotestosterone. A metabolite of testosterone involved in regulating sexual drive and the development of sexual organs. Essential for normal growth and development, normal sexual arousal and expansion of muscular tissue. Involved in hair and prostate growth. Found in skin, gums, hair follicles, prostate and the brain. Works the same way in men and women.

Dioxin. Tetrachlorodibenzodioxin. Also known as TTDD. An insecticide that kills plants and mosquitoes. Also known as "Agent Orange" in the Vietnam War. Produced as a by-product when chlorinated materials such as plastics are burned. Toxic at a dilution of less than one part per trillion. A proven cause of cancer, not merely statistically linked to a higher risk of cancer. A powerful hormone-disrupting chemical associated with a small penis, lowered sperm count, miscarriages and reproductive disorders including infertility.

DNA. Deoxyribonucleic acid. The blueprint of life. The coded information or blueprint for every living thing. A molecule of DNA in which nucleic acids are coiled in a helical structure has the ability to reproduce itself within the cell. Toxins, UV light, vitamin deficiencies and radiation can alter DNA. Several sections of the molecule have regulatory functions that can turn genes off and on.

Dopamine. The pleasure chemical that is able to bridge the gap (synapse) between neurons (nerve cells) and send signals from one neuron to another. Dopamine is essential for feeling pleasure. Insufficient amounts of dopamine can cause chronic fatigue, stimulate the appetite and interfere with concentration. Too much dopamine can induce hallucinations, aggressive behavior and excessive libido. Nicotine and testosterone both increase dopamine.

E2 or Estradiol. The "active" female estrogen. Secreted by the ovaries, testicles and adrenal glands. E2 is present in most birth control pills, female hormone supplements, patches and pills.

Endorphins. Natural morphine-like (opioid) chemicals in the brain. Can decrease the perception of pain, creating a state of euphoria, or feeling "high." They can be triggered by hormones, narcotics and exercise as well as by intense pain or pleasure.

Environmental estrogens or EDCs. Toxic compounds formed in the environment that mimic the function of the body's own estrogen compounds and are blamed for the deterioration and decrease in the number of human sperm, the decrease in reproduction of salmon, alligators, birds and other wildlife. Also termed xenoestrogens and endocrine disruptive chemicals.

Epinephrine Also known as adrenaline. Epinephrine is a powerful stimulant of female sexual arousal and increases heart rate, breathing and muscular strength.

Equilibrium dialysis. A sensitive test that has been developed to measure "free" (or circulating) levels of testosterone, about 2 to 4 percent of the total. Free testosterone when measured by *equilibrium dialysis*, provides a precise calculation of a man or woman's testosterone concentration.

Erogenous zones. Those parts of the body such nipples that respond to stimulation by becoming engorged with blood. Some areas contain erectile tissue. Erogenous stimulation is a precursor to sexual activity in all animals.

Estratest® Manufactured by Solvay, Belgium. The only combination estrogen-testosterone pill for women, which entered the market 20 years ago, but the FDA never approved it. It was finally approved in the past few years.

Estrogens. The three types, E1, E2 and E3, are known collectively as conjugated estrogens. In a healthy young adult female, the typical mix of these hormones is 10 to 20 percent estrone (E1), 10 to 20 percent estradiol (E2) and 60 to 80 percent estriol (E3). Estrogen stimulates the ovaries to make mature eggs and the testicles to make sperm. Estrogen promotes networking between brain cells by encouraging nerve development and blood flow to the brain.

Enzymes. Proteins formed by genes, which act as biological catalysts to aid in the manufacture of various bodily compounds. Enzymes are used for digestion, hormone conversion and tissue destruction. Some enzymes are triggered by light and can be marked with fluorescent dyes.

FDA. Food and Drug Administration. A government agency that regulates the use and safety of medicine. The FDA allows drugs to come to market but does not actually approve their use. Once approved, the manufacturer is allowed to sell the product on the open market without prosecution.

Free Testosterone or FT. A form of testosterone, which circulates freely in the body and is responsible for sexual function in both men and women. It comprises about 1–4% of the total testosterone.

FSD. Female sexual disorder. A new term for women who cannot achieve orgasm or have satisfactory sexual relations. Affects over 40 million women in the US and includes a wide range of sexual dysfunction.

FSH. Follicle stimulating hormone. A hormone that stimulates the developing egg and triggers its release from the ovary. At the same time it increases a woman's estrogen production it is involved in triggering the male testicles to grow.

GHRH. Growth hormone releasing hormone. A hormone originating in the hypothalamus, which regulates the secretion of the growth hormone during the night. It is only effective during deep rapid-eye-movement (REM) sleep.

Glycogen. A form of reserve of fat and muscle-stored sugars. Also found in the liver. Can be converted to glucose when energy is needed due to the action of a hormone in the pancreas.

Gynecomastia or gyno. Breast enlargement in males, usually occurring in adolescent males or in men using excess estrogen. Also referred to as man boobs, bitch tits or breast buds.

HCG. Human chorionic gonadotropin. A hormone produced early in pregnancy. Resembles LH in structure and so it can increase testosterone production by the cells in the testicles.

HGH. Human growth hormone. Short for recombinant human growth hormone. A protein molecule containing more than 190 amino acids which varies from species to species but is responsible for growth of muscle, bone and organs in all mammals. HGH levels peak in young adulthood and gradually taper off, therefore HGH is being sought after as an "anti-aging" drug.

HPA. Hypothalamus-pituitary-adrenal. The regulating system in the brain, located between the hypothalamus and the pituitary gland. The triangle of hormone interrelationships, the HPA begins to function poorly after a few months of constant, unremitting stress.

HRT. Hormone replacement therapy. Synthetic hormones, usually estrogen and progesterone, given to most women after menopause to replace hormones no longer made by their body.

Hypogonadism. Extremely low levels of testosterone, especially in the male but also in the female. Can be treated with testosterone replacement therapy if detected early. Usually refers to total testosterone levels of less than 300 nanograms per deciliter (ng/dl) in men or less than 3 ng/dl in women.

Hypothalamus. The hypothalamus is the seat of emotional expression and regulates everything from fear to aggression to sex drive. In addition to controlling hormonal functions, the body's water and salt balances, blood pressure, sugar and fat metabolism.

IGF-1. Insulin-like growth factor. A protein that regulates the secretion of GH and mimics the effect of insulin on the human body, making muscles more sensitive to the insulin effect. Circulating IGF-I levels increase at puberty to cause growth spurts and sex organ growth and then decrease to very low levels in the elderly.

Isoflavones. Hormone-like compounds found in soybeans. The main isoflavones are geneistin and daidzein. Isoflavones are a class of Phytoestrogens that are concentrated in soybeans. Soy isoflavones are also free radical scavengers (potent antioxidants) and are antiangiogenic (they interfere with unwanted blood vessel growth in disease states). Red clover leaves are purported to contain the highest amount of isoflavones.

Levitra® Manufactured by Bayer. Vardenafil. A new erection enhancing medication whose manufacturers claim has fewer side effects than Viagra. Levitra comes in 5, 10, 20 mg and enhances erections for about 4-6 hours.

LH. Luteinizing hormone. A hormone secreted by the pituitary gland to regulate the testicular production of testosterone and the ovarian production of progesterone or testosterone. LH may also be involved in regulating other hormonal releasing factors such as FSH and SHBG.

Lipitor®. Pfizer's best-selling anticholesterol agent. It regulates the liver's production of cholesterol and is used as a cholesterol-lowering drug for anyone with high cholesterol not responding to diet or hormone replacement.

Lithium or LithoBid. A very common basic element that is used as a mood stabilizer in persons with bipolar depression. Lithium can affect the thyroid gland and is effective in boosting the action of any antidepressant even in persons without bipolar depression.

Lycopenes. Antioxidants found in watermelon, grapes, tomatoes and some shellfish, released only by cooking the food. Lycopenes are one class of 650 carotenoids found in high concentrations in the testicles of normal males and in low levels in infertile males. Lycopenes have been used to help treat dioxin-induced infertility in men.

Mediterranean diet. A diet that eliminates red meat and uses large servings of fish, fresh vegetables, olive oil and pasta to control heart disease and reduce high cholesterol levels.

Melatonin. A hormone regulator released by the pineal gland in the brain, causing sleepiness and enabling one to fall asleep when it gets dark at night. Regulates the body's internal clock and the cycles of other hormones. Melatonin also regulates the action of other hormones.

Muscle Dysmorphia. An obsession with muscular development of the human body. Men with this condition think they are never "big enough" regardless of how much muscle mass they develop. This condition can lead to anabolic steroid abuse, obesity and premature death.

Muse® Made by Vivus. A prostaglandin derivative inserted into the end of the penis to induce an erection. Obviously, though it worked, it never became very popular. Now available as a cream injected into the urethra.

Natural opioids. Substances in nature, which impact the brain's receptors for pain and pleasure. Steroid hormones can induce beta-endorphins, the brain's own morphine-like compounds. These compounds can alter the perception of pain and pleasure. Opioid substances derived from the opium poppy can block these pain receptors.

Neurosteroids or neurohormones. Neurohormones are a fascinating class of hormones that are created in your brain's control center and serve as signaling, transmitting and switching devices. These chemical messengers are secreted from nerve cells or neurons. Neurosteroids are made in the brain from progesterone or pregnenolone. They can circulate in the blood stream or work locally on other brain cells.

Neurotransmitters. Molecules consisting of proteins, which carry the message from one nerve to another across a space- a "synapse" in the brain or spinal cord. They can also act as hormones and trigger the release of brain hormones. Neurotransmitters regulate our moods, our appetite, our sleeping, dreaming, impulses, energy levels and perception of pain.

NO. Nitric oxide. A gas that changes the walls of the blood vessels, swelling the arteries so that blood can fill the blood vessels. NO allows blood to flow into the penis and is increased by erections enhances like Viagra, Levitra and Cialis.

Norepinephrine or noradrenaline. A precursor of dopamine and an essential brain and spinal cord neurotransmitter. Norepinephrine (NE) is crucial for nerves to communicate and triggers arousal in men. NE can act as a hormone in the brain triggering other hormones involved in arousal.

NRIs. Norepinephrine reuptake inhibitors

Oxytocin. A sex hormone secreted by the pituitary, testicles, ovaries and the brain. Directs female nursing and birthing plus bonding behaviors in many animal species. May even play an important role in ejaculation, orgasm and sexual preference.

PASAS. Post anabolic steroid abuse syndrome. A collection of symptoms that occur in men, who have been self-medicating with anabolic steroids and then suddenly stop. Loss of erections is the first sign of PASAS, a term Dr. Kryger coined. This syndrome is not recognized by the AMA.

Pheromones. Humans use pheromones-odorless, chemical messages that we continuously emit through our skin-to communicate, protect our children and recognize and connect with each other, on what feels like an "intuitive" level. Pheromones may even explain why we feel comfortable with some people and have virtually nothing to say to other people; why we're attracted to some people and repulsed by others. They are totally different chemical compounds in men and women and companies have been unsuccessful in manufacturing them.

Phthalates. Dioxin-like chemicals routinely used in soaps, shampoos and nail polish and in medical products like tubing and plastics to keep them soft and flexible. Phthalates and dioxin exposure can have devastating effects on the developing sex organs of men and women.

Phytochemicals or phytonutrients. Beneficial antioxidants and other plant-based compounds. Vitamins C and E used in conjunction with the beneficial bioflavinoids from fresh fruits, seeds, nuts and vegetables can remove bioactive compounds which can cause the DNA and tissue damage.

Phytoestrogens. Plant-based compounds that can bind to the estrogen receptor without generating estrogen activity. By blocking this receptor they stop the occurrence of hot flashes, decrease bone loss and reduce the risk of breast cancer in some women. Phytoestrogens are hormone-like bioregulators that come from plants, without the harmful side effects related to some estrogens.

Pregnenelone. The most abundant hormone in the brain. Pregnenolone is a precursor for every other hormone. This hormone is the second step in the formation of all hormones from cholesterol. When used as a supplement, it seems to work as a neurotransmitter to clarify thinking, promote concentration and prevent memory loss.

Premarin® by Wyeth. A popular estrogen used in estrogen replacement programs. Derived from pregnant mare's urine (PREgnant MARe's urINe). The most popular conjugated estrogen in the world.

Progesterone. A hormone best known for its role in preparing the lining of the uterus to secure the placement of the fertilized egg, is also involved in the production of important hormones for both men and women. Progesterone physically opposes the action of estrogen in women just as testosterone opposes estrogen excess in men. It seems to affect SHBG levels and sexual drive in women and can convert easily to testosterone. In the brain, progesterone can act as a neurosteroid calming the individual.

Progestins. Sex hormones that are synthetic versions of progesterone, made in labs to last at least 24 hours in the body. Commonly combined with Premarin as Provera.

Prolactin. A hormone secreted by the pituitary gland. In women prolactin regulates the flow of milk from the breasts of nursing mothers; in men prolactin secreted after male ejaculation brings about a refractory period that prevents another erection for at least one half hour. Prolactin inhibits sexual desire in men and prolactin also causes women to feel less sexual desire after giving birth.

Prometrium® Manufactured by Solvay. A real progesterone form that is available in vaginal cream or oil filled capsule for women needing bioidentical progesterone supplementation.

Prostaglandin. Discovered in the prostate glands of sheep in 1982, they played a role in testosterone regulation through feedback to the pituitary gland. Injected directly into the penis of impotent men prostaglandins (Caverjet®) generates an immediate firm erection. Topical forms of Alprostadil® or Alprox® and Topiglan® are being developed by pharmaceutical companies.

Provera® Manufactured by Wyeth. A synthetic progesterone or progestin. May be the culprit in causing breast cancer and the side effects seen with hormone replacement therapy.

Provigil® Modafinil. Manufactured by Cephalon. An alertness drug that activates the brain's histamine system. Recently approved for jet lag and shift workers plus for narcolepsy and sleep disorders.

Psychotropic medications. Medicines that work in the mind such as tranquilizers, antidepressants, antipsychotics and stimulants, including street drugs like speed, methamphetamine, crack cocaine and legal drugs such as caffeine and nicotine.

PVN. Paraventricular nucleus. Located next to the hypothalamus. Creates oxytocin during sexual arousal.

Rozerem™ or Ramelteon. Manufactured by Takeda . A new class of hypnotics to induce sleep. This drug affects certain melatonin receptors (M1 and M2) and is approved for long-term use without incidence of withdrawal or dependence. It is the only non-controlled sleep aid on the market available by prescription.

SCN. Suprachiasmatic nucleus. The body's clock processing light signals and determining how much melatonin the pineal gland should release. Located in the brain inside the hypothalamus and produces vasopressin. The SCN may be the site of the sexually dimorphic nucleus, which determines sexual preference. The SCN is also loaded with receptors that are stimulated by oxytocin, which is released during ejaculation and orgasm.

Secondary hypogonadism. A condition of testosterone deficiency, which occurs later in life when the pituitary does not respond to low levels of testosterone by increasing its LH production.

Secretogogues. Amino acids that stimulate the pituitary and other organs of the body to release (secrete) hormones. An example is arginine, an amino acid that helps synthesize nitric oxide. L-arginine can stimulate the pituitary to secret human growth hormone for 45 minutes or so, but a pill with arginine in it has no such effect.

Serotonin syndrome. An overdose of serotonin (5-HT) can cause vomiting, loss of orientation and possibly death. Can occur when mixing SRIs with OTC products like St. John's Wort.

SDN. Sexually Dimorphic Nucleus of the Preoptic Area. A tiny area of the hypothalamus, which is larger in men than in women. It is important for developing sexual identity and behavior and it is extremely sensitive to sex hormones.

SHBG. Sex hormone binding globulin, SHBG increases with age, binding up more hormones and causing lower concentrations of biologically available testosterone. Also acts as a regulator of arousability in the hypothalamus and can turn sex hormones off and on.

SRIs or SSRIs. Specific Serotonin re-uptake inhibitors. A popular class of antidepressants including Prozac, Paxil®, Zoloft®, Lexapro® and Celexa®. These are very effective in treating severe premenstrual conditions and depression by affecting serotonin receptors.

Somatopause. A period from early adulthood onward when our pituitary gland releases less and less growth hormone, so we stop growing and start aging. Freud said that at age 35 we become aware of our own mortality; somatopause occurs much earlier.

Somatostatin. A biologic blocker of the growth hormone inhibiting hormone (GHIH) or (GHRH). Blocks the pituitary production of HGH and increases with aging.

Steroids. Compounds based on the "sterol" molecule from cholesterol. Also common terms referring to anabolic hormones that can increase muscle mass and are used by many bodybuilders to boost the size of their muscles. Most hormones are actually steroids.

T4. Thyroxine. The main hormone secreted by the thyroid gland. Thyroxine contains 4 iodine molecules and is converted to T3, the active form of thyroid hormone in the thyroid gland.

TCDD. Tetrachloro-dibenzo-dioxin. The most toxic dioxin found into the environment. As little as 5 parts per trillion can be lethal. TCDD is used interchangeably with dioxin in this book.

Testim®· Manufactured by Auxillium. A new 1% testosterone gel; released to market by the FDA in 2003. Auxillium claims that it is more potent than AndroGel and increases testosterone levels more effectively.

TestoDerm®. Manufactured by Alza. The first testosterone transdermal plastic patch applied to the scrotum. Although extremely effective it was discontinued, since it was too large and uncomfortable and did not sell well. No other testosterone product has been approved for application to the scrotum. Alza Pharmaceuticals was taken over by Johnson and Johnson in 2004.

Testosterone or T. The most important of the male hormones. A molecule originating in male and female sexual organs, circulating at different levels in men and women, normal total testosterone levels for adult males range from 300 to 1100 ng/dl or nanograms per deciliter. Testosterone influences men's ability to perform different types of tasks involving spatial memory, motivational tasks and is responsible for dominant behavior.

Testosterone cypionate. An injectable testosterone that lasts about 4 to 9 days. It is a moderately long-acting testosterone mixed with peanut oil for injection into the gluteus muscle.

Tribulus. An over-the-counter, purported testosterone stimulant, an herbal preparation. Tribulus has been found scientifically to have minimal effects on testosterone production.

TRT. Testosterone replacement therapy. A program of daily testosterone supplementation designed to improve man's sexual drive and moods as well as the firmness of the penis during sexual intercourse.

TSH. Thyroid stimulating hormone. TSH is released from the pituitary to stimulate the thyroid to secrete thyroxine or T4. TSH levels are used as a screening test for thyroid disorders. TSH has also been found to affect the formation of bone.

Vasopressin (VP). Also called anti-diuretic hormone or ADH. A neurohormone that originates in the pituitary gland and is involved in controlling nighttime urine production, sexual arousal and aggression and regulating the fluid volume of the body.

Wellbutrin®. Manufactured by Galaxo-Smith-Kline. A very safe and effective antidepressant used as a dopamine stimulant to help smokers quit smoking, decrease weight and increase sexual drive in women. Available in a new XL or long-lasting form as well as generic called Bupropion.

WHI. Women's Health Initiative. A study that put traditional hormone replacement therapy in a very bad light. Based on long-term studies over a quarter of a century involving thousands of women, the organization reported in 2002, that equine (horse) estrogens and synthetic progestins like Provera, did not protect women against heart disease but actually increased the risk of cancer, dementia and heart attacks. However, the study found that HRT did prevent osteoporosis and skin wrinkling.

WHO. World Health Organization. A global nonprofit organization that promotes sanitation, health initiatives and education for nutrition and physical health. This group tracks epidemics and pandemics.

Xenoestrogens (*xeno* is Greek for "stranger"). Estrogens derived from the environment and concentrated in the fat of animals used for food. These environmental estrogens, are affecting the fertility and sexual functions of all the world's citizens.

Yohimbine or Yocon®. An alpha receptor blocker that comes from the bark of a tree from Africa. Used by tribal witch doctors as a treatment for sexual problems. Once available as an over-the-counter male enhancement product, but now available only by prescription as Yocon®. Yocon is believed to work as a libido enhancer but studies using high doses have not confirmed this claim.

RESOURCES

Recommended Books

The following books were written for non-medical people who want to know more about their hormones, longevity and sexuality. I do not necessarily agree with everything in these books, but I think they are important for a solid background in the field of how your hormones affect your sexlife, your love life and your longevity.

Archer J, Lloyd B. *Sex and Gender* (2nd ed.). New York: Cambridge University Press. 2002

Berman J, Berman L. *For Women Only: A Revolutionary Guide to Overcoming Sexual Dysfunction and Reclaiming Your Sex Life.* Henry Holt and Company. 2001

Blasius M. (Ed.). *Sexual Identities, Queer Politics.* Princeton, NJ: Princeton University Press. 2001

Blum, Deborah. *Sex On The Brain.* New York: Penguin Putman Inc. 1997

Brown, Lester R. *Eco-Economy: Building an Economy for the Earth.* NY. W.W.Norton &Company. 2004

Burwash, Paul. *Total Health The Next Level: A Simple Guide for Taking Control of Your Health and Happiness Now!* Torchlight Publishing. 1997

Cadbury, Deborah, *The Estrogen Effect: How Chemical Pollution is Threatening Our Survival.* St. Martin's Press, NY. 1997

Calvin, William H.: *How Brains Think; Evolving Intelligence, Then and Now.* Harper Collins Publishers Inc. 1996

Carruthers, Malcolm. *The Testosterone Revolution.* Thorsons. 2000. Originally published as *The Male Menopause,* HarperCollins, 1996

Colborn, Theo, Dumanoski D, Myers JP. *Our Stolen Future, Are We Threatening Our Fertility, Intelligence and Survival? A Scientific Detective Story.* Plum (Penguin) 1997

D'Augelli A. R., & Patterson, C. J. (Eds.). *Lesbian, Gay and Bisexual Identities and Youth: Psychological Perspectives.* New York: Oxford University Press. 2001

Dean T. *Beyond Sexuality.* Chicago: University of Chicago Press. 2000

Diamond, Jed. *Surviving Male Menopause: A Guide for Women and Men.* Sourcebooks, Inc. 2000

Diamond J. *The Warrior's Journey Home.* New Harbinger Publications Inc. 1994

Diamond J. *Male Menopause.* Sourcebooks, Inc. 1997

Esterberg K. G. *Lesbian and Bisexual Identities: Constructing Communities, Constructing Selves.* Philadelphia, PA: Temple University Press. 1997

Fisher H. *Why We Love. The Nature and Future of Romantic Love.* Henry Holt and Co. Inc. 2004

Goldstein I. *Women's Sexual Function and Dysfunction: Study, Diagnosis and Treatment.* Informa Health Care/Taylor & Francis. 2006

Goodall Jane et al. *Harvest for Hope: A Guide to Mindful Eating.* 2005

Johnson Olive S. *The Sexual Spectrum. Exploring Human Diversity.* Vancouver, BC. RainCoast Books. 2004.

Hakim L, *The Couple's Disease: Finding a Cure for your Lost Love Life.* DHP Publishers, 2002

Hoberman, John. *Testosterone Dreams: Rejuvenation, Aphrodisia, Doping.* University of California Press. 2005

Kahn, Carol. *Beyond the Double Helix: DNA and the Quest for Longevity,* Times Books, 1985

Krimsky S. *Hormonal Chaos: The Scientific and Social Origins of the Environmental Endocrine Hypothesis.* The Johns Hopkins University Press. 2000

Kryger, Meir H. *The Woman's Guide to Sleep Disorders.* The McGraw-Hill Companies. 2004

Malesky G. Kittel M. *The Hormone Connection: Revolutionary Discoveries Linking Hormones and Women's Health Problems.* Prevention Health Books for Women. Rodale Inc. 2001

Manning, John. *Digit Ratio:* A Pointer to Fertility, Behavior and Health. Rutgers University Press, New Jersey 2002

Old J. *Vintage People: The Secrets of Successful Aging.* Pathway Publications. 2000

Patterson C. *Eternal Treblinka: Our Treatment of Animals and the Holocaust,* Lantern Books, NY 2002

Quinn D. M. *Same-sex Dynamics Among Nineteenth-Century Americans: A Mormon Example.* Urbana, IL: University of Illinois Press. 1996

Rako, Susan. *The Hormone of Desire.* Three Rivers Press, NY. 1996

Reid, DP. *The Tao of Health, Sex and Longevity: A Modern Practical Guide to the Ancient Way.* Fireside. 1989

Reiss I. L., Ellis, A. *At the Dawn of the Sexual Revolution: Reflections on a Dialogue.* Walnut Creek, CA: Altamira Press. 2002

Richardson D. *Rethinking Sexuality.* London: Sage Publications. 2000

Richardson D., & Seidman, S. (Eds.). *Handbook of Lesbian and Gay Studies.* London: Sage Publications. 2002

Robbins, John. *Diet for A New America: How Your Food Choices Affect your Health, Happiness and the Future of Life on Earth.* HJ Kramer. 1987

Robbins, John. *The Food Revolution: How Your Diet Can Help Save Your Life and the World.* Conari Press, Berkeley, California. 2001

Robbins, John. *Reclaiming Our Health: Exploding the Medical Myth and Embracing the Source of True Healing.* HJ Kramer Inc. 1996

Schechter A, Gasiewicz TA. *Dioxins and Health,* second edition. John Wiley & Sons, 2003

Shippen, Gene, Fryer William. *The Testosterone Syndrome. The Critical Factor For Energy, Health, & Sexuality: Reversing The Male Menopause.* M. Evans and Company. 1998

Somers, Suzanne. *The Sexy Years: Discover The Hormone Connection.* Crown Publishers, NY. 2004

Thomas C. (Ed.). *Straight with a Twist: Queer theory and the Subject of Heterosexuality.* Urbana, IL: University of Illinois Press. 2000

Thornton J. *Pandora's Poison: Chlorine, Health and a New Environmental Strategy.* MIT Press. 2000

Townsend J.M. *What Women Want, What Men Want: Why the Sexes Still See Love and Commitment so Differently.* New York: Oxford University Press. 1998

Veldhuis J, Iranmanesh A, Mulligan T. *Toward a Healthier Old Age: Biomedical Advances from Basic Research to Clinical Science.* Barcelona, Spain: Prous Science Publishers. 1999

Weil Andres. *Healthy Aging: A Lifelong Guide to Your Physical and Spiritual Well-Being.* Alfred A Knopf, New York. 2005

Willcox Bradley, Willcox Craig, Suzuki M. *The Okinawa Program.* NY: Three Rivers Press. 2001

Helpful Information from the Worldwide Web
(Be forewarned, some of these links may be offline)

Adult Growth Hormone Replacement. Key points by the Society of Endocrinology on diagnosing and treating adults with a deficiency of somatrophin or growth hormone at: www.endocrinology.org/SFE/gh.htm

American Association of Clinical Endocrinologists (AACE). For press releases on professional meetings, new studies and reports on research in the field of endocrinology, go to: www.aace.com/pub/press/releases

For current guidelines regarding medication and other treatment of hormone-related disorders, go to www.aace.com/clin/guidelines

Andropause. Information by the Canadian andropause Society, at the location: www.andropause.com

Anabolic Steroid Abuse. National Institute on Drug Abuse. A government program dealing with problems and solutions involving the misuse of steroids, www.steroidabuse.org

Androglogy Database: Normal male hormone ranges for animals and humans, http://www.il-st-acad-sc.org/data3.html

Cannabis. Health Aspects and changes in male sex hormones. A 1986 paper provided by the American Society of Pharmacology and Experimental Therapies, http://www.users.lycaeum.org/~painter/ENDWAR/marij1.html

Control of Endocrine Activity. An illustrated presentation from Colorado State University on how the body regulates the supply and delivery of hormones at: http://arbl.cvmbs.colostate.edu/hbooks/pathphys/endocrine/basics/control.html

Endocrine System Topics. For comprehensive reports from the National Institutes of health, go to the following URL and enter the word or words in the search box at the top of the page. www.nlm.nih.gov/medicineplus/search.html

Endocrinology of Aging. Easy to understand discussion of current thinking on aging and hormones. The report was financed by Soreno, a leading biotech research firm. Go to: www.medscape.com/viewarticle/407921_1

Endocrinology Glossary of Patient Conditons. The medical school at the University of Maryl and has prepared a readable glossary of key terms related to hormones at: http://www.umm.edu/endocrin/glossary.htm

Endocrine Disorders of Patients. The treatment through surgery of hormones glands such as thyroid and adrenal from benign and malignant tumors as well as hormone and metabolic responses to surgery. http://www.umm.edu/general_surgery/pat_cond.html

Estradiol. The Aeron Saliva testing lab gives normal levels of this hormone for males and females at the location: http://www.aeron.com/estradiol.htm

Estrogen Evolution. The Hormone Foundation, a public education organization of the Endocrine Society, provides helpful links about the use and misuse of hormones. Go to the home page at: www.hormone.org and enter "estrogen" in the search box at the top of the screen.

FDA CenterWatch. Drugs Approved by the FDA (search by name). www.centerwatch.com

Genetic Testing and Counseling. Enter key words in the search box for pages on this topic, provided by the National Institutes of Health, at www. nlm.nih.gov

GH Use in Adults and Children. Guidelines for prescribing growth hormone, from the American Association of Clinical Endocrinologists at the location: http://www.aace.com/clin/guidelines/hgh.pdf

Growth Hormone (GH) Replacement in Older Men. Comprehensive information by eMedicine, at: www.emedicine.com/med/topic3178.htm

Hormone Chemistry and Synthesis. Good textbook explanation provided by Colorado State University of how hormones work in the human body, at: arbl.cvmbs.colostate.edu/hbooks/pathphys/endocrine/basics/chem

Hormone Rhythms. Brief patient information on topics selected by the Endocrine Society. Go to: www.endo-society.org/pubrelations/news.cfm and enter "hormone rhythms" in the search box.

Hormones of the Reproductive System. A comprehensive illustrated discussion of hormones of the reproductive system at users.rcn.com/jkimball.ma.ultranet/BiologyPages/S/SexHormones.html

Hormones, Receptors and Target Cells. Easy to understand information from Colorado State University. Go to: arbl.cvmbs.colostate.edu/hbooks/pathphys/endocrine/basics/ hormones.html

Male Hormones Linked to Prostate Cancer. Personal MD offers information to the general public on a variety of topics. Enter key words in the search box at www.personalmd.com

Mechanisms of Hormone Action. Great textbook discussion by Colorado State University at: arbl.cvmbs.colostate.edu/hbooks/pathphys/endocrine/moaction/index.html

Menopausal Hormone Replacement Therapy (HRT). Provided for the general public at by the National Cancer Institute www.meb.uni-bonn.de/cancernet/600310.html

Menopause Online. Information for the general public on the menopause at www.menopause-online.com

Neuroendocrine System: Pituitary and Hypothalamus. Illustrated textbook information by Colorado State University, at the location: arbl.cvmbs.colostate.edu/hbooks/pathphys/endocrine/hypopit/overview.html

Pituitary Axis. Information about the hypothalamus and pituitary gland by Colorado State University at the location: arbl.cvmbs.colostate.edu/hbooks/pathphys/endocrine/hypopit/index.html

Sex Hormone Tests. HealthyMe gives normal levels of all sex hormones www.ahealthyme.com/topic/topic100587459.htm

Sexual Reproduction in Humans. Full-color illustrations and text, at: users.rcn.com/jkimball.ma.ultranet/BiologyPages/S/Sexual_Reproduction. html#Spermatogenesis

Testosterone, Free and Weakly Bound: Serum Measurements. Technical data by the Laboratory Corporation of America, at: www.labcorp.com/datasets/labcorp/html/chapter/mono/sr016000.html

U.S. Food and Drug Administration (FDA). Information about how the FDA regulates drugs in the US, at: www.fda.gov/cder/drug/default.html

Women's Health Initiative (WHI). Details about the Women's Health Initiative research project about the use of estrogen in hormone replacement therapy. Go to: www.whi.org

Videos and Books on Tape

Klapper, Michael K. Pregnancy, *Children and the Vegan Diet. Vegan Nutrition. A Diet for All Reasons* (video) 1996. www.EarthSave.com

Kryger, Abraham H. *Listen To Your Hormones.* CD and MP3 files at the location: www.naturalecho.com and www.audible.com . www.book.google. com

Robbins, John. Diet for a New America. (video). Available at the location: www.foodrevolution.org

Weil Andrew. *Eating Well For Optimum Health: The Essential Guide to Bringing Health and Pleasure Back to Eating* (Audio-Unabridged). 1998.

Email Consultation Service

DrK@WellnessMD.com

Abraham Harvey Kryger, MD, DMD, the Wellness MD. Confidential and secure email consultations—medical subjects only at:
www.kryger.medem.com

Resources

Products and Services Mentioned in this Book

Diamond Organics, Inc.
Highway 1, Moss Landing, California 95039
1-888-ORGANIC (888-674-2642)
www.diamondorganics.com

Earthbound Farm
1721 San Juan Highway
San Juan Bautista, California 95045
www.ebfarm.com

Earthbound Farm's Farm Stand
7250 Carmel Valley Road
Carmel, California 93923
831-625-6219
e-mail farmstand@ebfarm.com

Full Spectrum Light Box
Northern Light Technologies
8971 Henri-Bourassa W.
Montreal, Canada H4S 1P7
800-263-0066
www.northernlight-tech.com

Gourmet Mushrooms, Inc.
2901 Granvenstein Highway North
Sebastopol, California 95472
707 823-1743, fax: 707-823-1507
www.mycopia.com

Immune Stimulating Mushrooms
Mycology Research Labs
Brough, East Yorkshire
United Kingdom HU15 1EF
http://mycologyresearch.com or www.aneid.com

Juice Plus+ natural, organic fruit and vegetable capsules
NSA
Memphis TN, 38118
www.juiceplus.com/+ak87117

Omega Fish Liver Oils
Nordic Naturals Inc.
Watsonville, California
831-724-6200
www.nordicnaturals.com

Pure Grapeseed Oil
Soofer Company, Inc.
Los Angeles Calif. 90058
800 852-4050 extension 120
www.sadaf.com

Smart Balance™ Tasty Butter Substitute
GFA Br ands Inc.
Heart Beat Foods Division
PO Box 397
Cresskill, NJ 07626
www.smartbalance.com

Estrocreme®, Testocreme®, TestoJel®
Websites for information about bioidentical hormone creams:
www.Testocreme.com
www.Estrocreme.com
www.TestoJel.com

HeartBars Plus ™
Unither Pharma
1077 Highway A1A
Satellite Beach, FL 32937
www.unitherpharma.com

Promensil™
Novogen Inc
One Landmark Square, 2nd Floor
Stamford, CT 06901
203-327-1188
www.promensil.com

Remifemin®
Enzymatic Therapy, Inc.
825 Challenger Drive
Green Bay, WI 54311
www.remifemin.com

WellnessMD Publications
1084 Cass Street-Suite B
Monterey, California. 93940
831 373-4406
Fax 831 373-4481
www.WellnessMD.com
www.sexloveandhormones.com
wellnessmd@earthlink.net

Sources for Information Included in this Book

The following medical and scientific resources were valuable to me in preparing this book. Most of the references are available on PubMed at the location: (http://www.ncbi.nlm.nih.gov/entrez/query.fcgi).

You will find them of special interest if you are familiar with medical research and literature. I have organized the references under topics covered as a bibliography.

Depression, Stress and Testosterone
Boschert S. Approvals Near for New Antidepressant Therapies. Family Practice News. Dec 1, 2002; 49

Booth A, Johnson DR, Granger DA. Testosterone and men's depression: the role of social behavior. J Health Soc Behav 1999 Jun;40(2):130-40

Carmin CN, Klocek JW. To screen or not to screen: symptoms identifying primary care medical patients in need of screening for depression. Int J Psychiatry Med 1998;28(3):293-302

Charmandari E, Kino T, Souvatzoglou E, Chrousos GP. Pediatric stress: hormonal mediators and human development. Horm Res 2003;59(4):161-79

Consoli SM. [Depression and associated organic pathologies, a still underestimated comorbidity. Results of the DIALOGUE study] [Article in French] Presse Med 2003 Jan 11;32(1):10-21)

deKloet ER. Stress in the brain. Eur J Pharm 2000,Sep 29;405:1-3; 187-98

Goodyer IM, Park RJ, Netherton CM, Herbert J. Possible role of cortisol and dehydroepiandrosterone in human development and psychopathology. Br J Psychiatry 2001 Sep;179:243-9

Goodyer IM, Herbert J, Tamplin A, Altham PM. First-episode major depression in adolescents. Affective, cognitive and endocrine characteristics of risk status and predictors of onset. Br J Psychiatry 2000 Feb;176:142-9

Grossi AM, Zajecka J. *Critical Breakthroughs* in the Advancement of Depression Treatment. Quarter Four 2002.

Harris TO, et al. Morning cortisol as a risk factor for subsequent major depressive disorder in adult women. Br J Psychiatry 2000 Dec;177:505-10

Herbert J. Neurosteroids, brain damage and mental illness. Exp Gerontology.1998 Nov-Dec;33(7-8):713-27

Hirschfeld RM, Lewis L, Vornik LA. Perceptions and impact of bipolar disorder: how far have we really come? Results of the national depressive and manic-depressive association 2000 survey of individuals with bipolar disorder. J Clin Psychiatry 2003 Feb;64(2):161-74

Hunt PJ, et al. Improvement in mood and fatigue after dehydroepiandrosterone replacement in Addison's disease in a r andomized, double blind trial. J Clin Endocrinol Metab 2000 Dec;85(12):4650-6

Kuhn KU, et al. Chronic course and psychosocial disability caused by depressive illnesses in general practice patients during a one year period.

Michael A, Jenaway A, Paykel ES, Herbert J. Altered salivary dehydroepi androsterone levels in major depression in adults. Biol Psychiatry 2000 Nov 15;48(10):989-95

Narrow WE, Rae DS, Robins LN, et al. Revised prevalence estimates of mental disorders in the US: using a clinical significance criterion to reconcile two survey's estimates. Arch Gen Psychiatry 2002;62(6):5-9)

Ohata H, Arai K, Shibasaki T. Effect of chronic administration of a CRF(1) receptor antagonist, CRA1000, on locomotor activity and endocrine responses to stress. Eur J Pharmacol 2002 Dec 20;457(2-3):201-6

Osran H, Reist C, Chen CC, Lifrak ET, Chicz-DeMet A, Parker LN.Adrenal androgens and cortisol in major depression. Am J Psychiatry 1993 May;150(5):806-9

Pope HG Jr, Cohane GH, Kanayama G, Siegel AJ, Hudson JI. Testosterone gel supplementation for men with refractory depression: a r andomized, placebo-controlled trial. Am J Psychiatry 2003 Jan;160(1):105-11)

Rothermund K, Brandtstadter J. Depression in later life: cross-sequential patterns and possible determinants. Psychol Aging 2003 Mar;18(1):80-90

Sapolsky R. Why Stress Is Bad for Your Brain. 1999 Personal communication from Department of Biological Sciences, Stanford University, Stanford, CA 94305, USA.

Schweiger U, et al. Testosterone, Gonadotropin and Cortisol Secretion in Male Patients With Major Depression. Psychosomatic Medicine 1999; 61:292-296

Seidman SN, Spatz E, Rizzo C, Roose SP. Testosterone replacement therapy for hypogonadal men with major depressive disorder: a r andomized, placebo-controlled clinical trial. J Clin Psychiatry 2001 Jun;62(6):406-12

Serby M, Yu M. Overview: depression in the elderly. Mt Sinai J Medicine 2003 Jan;70(1):38-44

Shors TJ, Leuner B. Estrogen-mediated effects on depression and memory formation in females. J Affect Disord 2003 Mar;74(1):85-96

Singh RB, Kartik C, Otsuka K, Pella D, Pella J. Brain-heart connection and the risk of heart attack. Biomed Pharmacother 2002;56: 2:257-65.

Stamp J, Herbert J. Corticosterone modulates autonomic responses and adaptation of central immediate-early gene expression to repeated restraint stress. Neuroscience 2001;107(3):465-79

Thapar A, McGuffin P. A twin study of depressive symptoms in childhood. British Journal of Psychiatry 1994 Aug;165(2):259-65

van Niekerk JK, Huppert FA, Herbert J. Salivary cortisol and DHEA: association with

measures of cognition and well-being in normal older men and effects of three months of DHEA supplementation. Psychoneuroendocrinology 2001 Aug;26(6):591-612

Viau V, Meaney MJ. The inhibitory effect of testosterone on hypothalamic-pituitary-adrenal responses to stress is mediated by the medial preoptic area. Neurosci 1996 Mar 1;16(5):1866-76.

Wolkowitz OM, et. al. Double-blind treatment of major depression with DHEA or dehydroepi androsterone. Am J Psychiatry 1999 Apr;156(4):646-9.

Weiller E, Lecrubier Y, Maier W, Ustun TB. The relevance of recurrent brief depression in primary care. A report from the WHO project on Psychological Problems in General Health Care conducted in 14 countries. Eur Arch Psychiatry Clin Neurosci 1994;244(4):182-9

Drugs and Testosterone

English KM, Pugh PJ, Parry H, Scutt NE, Channer KS, Jones The effect of cigarette smoking on levels of bioavailable testosterone in healthy men. Clin Sci (Lond) 2001 Jun;100(6):661-5

Fazio SB, Mukamal, KJ. Alcohol Consumption and Coronary Heart Disease: What Do the Lessons of Hormone Replacement Therapy Teach Us?

Journal COM 2002 Dec;9(12):691-95

Field AE, Colditz GA, Willett WC, Longcope C, McKinlay JB. The relation of smoking, age, relative weight and dietary intake to serum adrenal steroids, sex hormones and sex hormone-binding globulin in middle-aged men. J Clin Endocrinol Metab 1994 Nov;79(5):1310-6

Finch PM, et al. Hypogonadism in patients treated with intrathecal morphine. Clin J Pain 2000 Sep;16(3):251-4

Iribarren C. Cigars pose serious risks; Modern Medicine 1998, April (66); 11

Kovacs EJ, Messingham KA. Influence of alcohol and gender on immune response. Alcohol Res Health. 2002;26(4):257-63.

Purohit V, Ahluwahlia BS, Vigersky RA. Marihuana inhibits dihydrotestosterone binding to the androgen receptor. Endocrinology 1980 Sep;107(3):848-50

Roberts LJ, Finch PM, Pullan PT, Bhagat CI, Price LM. Sex hormone suppression by intrathecal opioids: a prospective study. Clin J Pain 2002 May-Jun;18(3):144-8

Sauer WH, et al. Cigarette yield and the risk of myocardial infarction in smokers. Arch Intern Med 2002;162:300-306

Sparrow D, Bosse R, Rowe JW. The influence of age, alcohol consumption and body build on gonadal function in men. J Clin Endocrinol Metab 1980 Sep;51(3):508-12

Trueb RM. Association between Smoking and Hair Loss: Another Opportunity for Health Education against Smoking? Dermatology 2003;206(3):189-91

Endocrine Disruptive Chemicals

Ashida H. Suppressive effects of flavinoids on dioxin toxicity. Biofactors 2000;12(1-4):201-6

Bagchi D, et al. Free radicals and grape seed proanthocyanidin extract: importance in human health and disease prevention. Toxicology 2000 Aug 7;148(2 3):187-97

Burton JE, Michalek JE, Rahe AJ. Serum dioxin, chloracne and acne in veterans of Operation Ranch H and. Arch Environ Health 1998 May;53(3):199-204

Cadbury D, The Estrogen Effect: How chemical pollution is threatening our survival. St. Martin's Press, NY. 1997

Colborn T, Dumanoski D, Myers JP, Our Stolen Future, Are We Threatening Our Fertility, Intelligence and Survival? A Scientific Detective Story. Plum (Penguin) 1997.

Egel and GM, et al. Total Serum Testosterone and Gonadotropins in Workers Exposed to Dioxin. Am J Epidem 1994; 139 (3): 272-81.

Feeley M, Brouwer A. Health risks to infants from exposure to PCBs, PCDDs and PCDFs. Food Addit Contam 2000 Apr;17(4):325-33. mark-feeley@hc-sc.gc.ca

Fleming LE, Bean JA, Rudolph M, Hamilton K. Mortality in a cohort of licensed pesticide applicators in Florida. Occup Environ Med. 1999 Jan;56(1):14-21.

Gray LE Jr, Ostby J, Monosson E, Kelce WR. Environmental anti androgens: low doses of the fungicide vinclozolin alter sexual differentiation of the male rat. Toxicol Ind Health 1999 Jan;15(1-2):48-64

Gray LE Jr. Xenoendocrine disrupters: laboratory studies on male reproductive effects. Toxicol Lett 1998 Dec 28;102-103:331-335

Harder B. Moms', Pops', sons' problems: Testicular cancer tied to a fetus' pollutant contact. Science News 2003;163/2/22.

Johnson L, et al. Reduced Leydig cell volume and function in adult rats exposed to 2,3,7,8-TCDD without a significant effect on spermatogenesis. Toxicology 1992 Nov 30;76(2):103-18

Krimsky S, Hormonal Chaos: The Scientific and Social Origins of the Environmental Endocrine Hypothesis. The Johns Hopkins University Press, 2000.

Mehta J, et al. Maternal exposure to a low dose of 2,3,7,8- TCDD suppressed the development of reproductive organs of male rats: dose-dependent increase of mRNA levels of 5alpha-reductase type 2 in contrast to decrease of androgen receptor in the pubertal ventral prostate. Toxicol Sci 2001 Mar;60(1):132-43

Morgan K. Hormones: Here's the Beef. Environmental concerns reemerge over steroids given to livestock. Science News. Jan 5, 2002;161:10-11

Morgantaler A. Toxins in People. Journal of the American Medical Assoc. April 15, 1998

Murray TJ, et al. Endocrine disrupting chemicals: Effects on human male reproductive health. Early Pregnancy 2001. Apr;5(2):80-112

Roberts J. US scientists class dioxins as a 'health concern'. BMJ 1994 Sep 24; 309 (6957):759-760

Rowlands JC, Gustafsson JA. Aryl hydrocarbon receptor-mediated signal transduction. Critical Review of Toxicology 1997 Mar;27(2):109-34

Sweeney MH, Calvert GM, Egel and GA, Fingerhut MA, Halperin WE, Piacitelli LA. Review and update of the results of the NIOSH medical study of workers exposed to chemicals contaminated with 2,3,7,8-tetrachlorodibenzodioxin. (TTCD).Teratog Carcinog Mutagen 1997-98;17(4-5):241-7

Thornton J. Pandora's Poison : Chlorine, Health and a New Environmental Strategy. MIT Press, 2000.

Watanabe S, et al. Effects of dioxins on human health: a review. J Epidemiol 1999 Feb;9(1):1-13

Whorton D, Krauss RM, Marshall S, Milby TH. Infertility in male pesticide workers. Lancet 1977 Dec 17;2(8051):1259-61

Females, DHEA and Testosterone Levels

Arlt W, et. al. Dehydroepi androsterone replacement in women with adrenal insufficiency. N Engl J Med 1999 Sep 30;341(14):1013-20

Bachmann G, et al. Female androgen insufficiency: the Princeton consensus statement on definition, classification and assessment. Fertil Steril. 2002 Apr;77(4):660-5.

Bancroft J, Davidson DW, Warner P, Tyrer G. androgens and sexual behaviour in women using oral contraceptives. Clinical Endocrinology. 1980;12:327-40.

Boehnert CE, Alberts RA. Seasonal Affective Disorder in Women: How to identify and treat. Postgraduate Medicine. 2003 Jan; 6 (1): 32-36.

Davis SR. Recent advances in female sexual dysfunction. Current Psychiatry Rep 2000 Jun;2(3):211-4

Davis SR. Testosterone deficiency in women. J Reprod Med 2001 Mar;46(3):291-6. Suedavis@netlink.com.au

*Mohr B, Guay AT, O'Donnell AB, McKinlay JB, Morley JE, et al. Normal, bound and nonbound testosterone levels in normally ageing men: results from the Massachusetts Male Ageing Study. Clinical Endocrinology (2005) 62: 64-73. BethM@neri.org

*Davison SL, R Bell R, Donath S, Montalto JG , Davis SR. androgen levels in adult females: changes with age. Journal of Clinical Endocrinology & Metabolism. First published April 12, 2005

Labrie F, Belanger A, Cusan L, Candas B . Physiological changes in DHEA (dehydroepi androsterone) are not reflected by serum levels of active androgens and estrogens but of their metabolites: intracrinology. J Clin Endocrinol Metab 1997 Aug;82(8):2403-9

Maleskey Gale, Kittel Mary. The Hormone Connection: Revolutionary Discoveries Linking Hormones and Women's Health Problems. Rodale Inc. St. Martin's Press. 2001

Modelska K, Cummings S. Female sexual dysfunction in postmenopausal women: systematic review of placebo-controlled trials. Am J Obstet Gynecol.2003;188: 286-293.

Morales AJ, Nolan JJ, et al. Effects of replacement dose of DHEA in men and women of advancing age. Journal of Clinical Endocrinology & Metabolism.1994;78:1360 7.

Rako S. Testosterone supplemental therapy after hysterectomy with or without concomitant oophorectomy: estrogen alone is not enough. J Women's Health Gend Based Med. 2000 Oct;9(8):917-23. Susanrako@aol.com

Rako S. Testosterone deficiency: a key factor in the increased cardiovascular risk to women following hysterectomy or with natural aging? J Women's Health. 1998 Sep;7(7):825-9.

Rako S. Testosterone deficiency and supplementation for women: What do we need to know? Menopause Management, September/October. GCS Press, LLC. 1996;5:10-15.

Randolph, JF Jr, MD, Dennerstein, L. Female androgen Deficiency Syndrome: A Hard Look at a Sexy Issue. Medscape Women's Health 6(2), 2001. 2001 Medscape, Inc

Rivera-Woll LM, Papalia M, Davis SR, et al. androgen insufficiency in women: diagnostic and therapeutic implications. Hum Reprod Update. 2004;10:421-432.

Sherwin BB, Gell and MM, Brender W. androgen enhances sexual motivation in females: a prospective cross-over study of sex steroid administration in the surgical menopause. Psychosomatic Med 1985;47:339-51

Shifren JL. Androgen deficiency in the oophorectomized woman. Fertil Steril. 2002 Apr;77 Suppl 4:S60-2.

Silva PD, Gentzschein EE, Lobo RA. Androstenedione may be a more important precursor of tissue dihydrotestosterone than testosterone in women. Fertility & Sterility 1987 Sep;48(3):419-22

Van Goozen SH, Wiegant VM, Endert E, Helmond FA, Van de Poll NE. Psychoendocrinological assessment of the menstrual cycle: the relationship between hormones, sexuality and mood. Arch Sex Behav 1997 Aug;26(4):359-82

Zofkova I, Zajickova K, Hill M, Horinek A. Apolipoprotein E gene determines serum testosterone and dehydroepi androsterone levels in postmenopausal women. Eur J Endocrinol 2001 Feb;147(4):503-506

Growth Hormone Information

Allen NE, et al. The associations of diet with serum insulin-like growth factor I and its main binding proteins in 292 women meat-eaters, vegetarians and vegans. Cancer Epidemiol Biomarkers Prev. 2002 Nov;11(11):1441-8.

Aimaretti G, Corneli G, Razzore P, et al. Comparison between insulin-induced hypoglycemia and growth hormone (GH)-releasing hormone + Arginine as provocative tests for the diagnosis of GH deficiency in adults. J Clin Endocrinol Metab 1998;83:1615

Appleby PN, Davey GK, Key TJ. Hypertension and blood pressure among meat eaters, fish eaters, vegetarians and vegans in EPIC-Oxford. Public Health Nutr. 2002 Oct;5(5):645-54.

Bhasin S, et al. Hormonal effects of GnRH agonist in the human male: II. Testosterone enhances gonadotrophin suppression induced by GnRH agonist. Clin Endocrinol (Oxf) 1984 Feb;20(2):119-28

Baum HB, et al. Effects of physiologic growth hormone therapy on bone density and body composition in patients with adult-onset of growth hormone deficiency. Ann Intern Med 1996;125:883-90.

Blackman MR, et al. Growth hormone and sex steroid administration in healthy aged women and men: a randomized controlled trial. JAMA 2002;288:2282-92.

Belgorosky A, et al. High serum sex hormone-binding globulin (SHBG) and low serum non-SHBG-bound testosterone in boys with idiopathic hypopituitarism: effect of recombinant human growth hormone treatment. Journal of Clinical Endocrinology & Metabolism. 1987 Dec;65(6):1107-11

Carani C, et al. The effect of chronic treatment with GH on gonadal function in men with isolated GH deficiency. Eur J Endocrinology 1999 Mar;140(3):224-30

Carroll P, Christ E. Growth hormone deficiency in adulthood and the effects of growth hormone replacement: a review. Journal of Clinical Endocrinology & Metabolism. 1998;83:382-95.

Deijen JB. van der Veen EA. The influence of growth hormone (GH) deficiency and GH replacement on quality of life in GH-deficient patients. Journal of Endocrinological Investigation.1999; 22(5):127-36.

Fazio S, Sabatini D, Capaldo B, et al A preliminary study of growth hormone in the treatment of dilated cardiomyopathy. New England J Medicine 1996;334:809-14.

Fisker S, Jorgensen JO, Christiansen JS. Variability in growth hormone stimulation tests. Growth Hormone, IGF Research 1998 Feb;8 (A):31-35

Fruchtman Sm Gift B, Howes B, Borski R. Insulin-like growth factor-I augments prolactin and inhibits growth hormone release through distinct as well as overlapping cellular signaling pathways. Comp Biochem Physiol B Biochem Mol Biol. 2001 Jun;129(2-3):237-42.

Gentili A, et al. Unequal impact of short-term testosterone repletion on the somatotropic axis of young and older men. Journal of Clinical Endocrinology & Metabolism. 2002 Feb;87(2):825-34.

Gibney J, et al. The effects of 10 years of recombinant human growth hormone (GH) in adult GH-deficient patients. Journal of Clinical Endocrinology & Metabolism. 1999 Aug; 84(8):2596-602.

Gomberg-Maitl and M, Frishman WH. Recombinant growth hormone: a new cardiovascular drug therapy. Am Heart J 1996;132:1244 -62.

Grimberg A, Cohen P. Role of insulin-like growth factors and their binding proteins in growth control and carcinogenesis. J Cell Physiol. 2000 Apr;183(1):1-9.

Guistina A, Lorusso R, Borghetti V, Bugari G, Misitano V, Alfieri O. Impaired spontaneous growth hormone secretion in severe dilated cardiomyopathy. Am Heart J 1996;131:620-22.

Hoffman D, O'Sullivan AJ, Baxter RC, Ho KKY. Diagnosis of growth-hormone deficiency in adults. Lancet 1994;343:1064-68.

Johannsson G, et al. Two years of growth hormone (GH) treatment increases bone mineral content and density in hypopituitary patients with adult-onset GH deficiency. J Clin Endocrin and Metab 1996;81:2865-73.

Johnston DG, et al. Long-term effects of growth hormone therapy on intermediary metabolism and insulin sensitivity in hypopituitary adults. Journal of Endocrinological Investigation. 1999; 22(5 Suppl):37-40.

Kim KR, et al. Low-dose GH treatment with diet restriction accelerates body fat loss, exerts anabolic effect and improves growth hormone secretory dysfunction in obese adults. Hormone Research.1999; 51(2):78-84.

Lamberts S, van den Beld A, van der Lely A. The endocrinology of aging. Science. 1997;278:419-424.

Leifke et al. Age-related changes of serum sex hormones, IGF-1 and SHBG levels in men: cross-sectional data from a healthy male cohort. Clin Endocrinology (Oxf) 2000 Dec;53(6):689-95.

Maison P, et al. Growth hormone as a risk for premature mortality in healthy subjects: data from the Paris prospective study. BMJ 1998 Apr 11;316(7138):1132-33.

Merimee TJ, Zapf J, Hewlett B, Cavalli-Sforza LL. Insulin-like growth factors in pygmies. The role of puberty in determining final stature. New England Journal of Med. 1987 Apr 9;316(15):906-11.

Patek SM, 1998 - AACE Guidelines for clinical practice for the evaluation and treatment of hypogonadism in adult male patients. Hypogonadism Task Force. Endocr Pract. 1996; 2:440-453) at: www.acce.com/clin/ guidelines/ hypogonadism.pdf

Papadakis MA, et al. Growth hormone replacement in older men improves body composition but not functional ability. Ann Intern Med 1996;124:708-716.

Rudman D, et al. Effects of human growth hormone in men over 60 years old. N Engl J Med 1990;323:1-6.

Taaffe DR, et al. Effect of recombinant human growth hormone on the muscle strength response to resistance exercise in elderly men. J Clinical Endocrinol Metab 1994;79:1361-66.

Savine R, Sonksen PH. Is the somatopause an indication for growth hormone replacement? J of Endocrinological Investigation. 1999;22(5 Suppl):142-9.

Shim M. IGFs and Human Cancer: Implications Regarding the Risk of Growth Hormone Therapy. Horm Res 1999, Nov; (51) S3:42-51.

Silva ME, et al. Effects of testosterone on growth hormone secretion and somatomedin-C generation in prepubertal growth hormone deficient male patients. Braz J Med Biol Res. 1992;25(11):1117-26.

Span JP, et al. Gender difference in insulin-like growth factor I response to growth hormone (GH) treatment in GH-deficient adults: role of sex hormone replacement. J Clin Endocrinol Metab 2000 Mar;85(3):1121-5.

Su HY, Hickford JG, Bickerstaffe R, Palmer BR. Insulin-like growth factor 1 and hair growth. Dermatol Online J. 1999 Nov;5(2):1.

Waters DL, Yau CL, Montoya GD, Baumgartner RN. Serum Sex Hormones, IGF-1 and IGFBP3 Exert a Sexually Dimorphic Effect on Lean Body Mass in Aging. J Gerontol A Biol Sci Med Sci. 2003 Jul;58(7):648-52.

Vance, M. L. Can Growth Hormone Prevent Aging?. New England Journal of Medicine 2003; 348: 779-780.

Measuring Testosterone

Belgorosky A, Rivarola MA. Changes in serum sex hormone-binding globulin and in serum non-sex hormone-binding globulin-bound testosterone during prepuberty in boys. J Steroid Biochem 1987;27(1-3):291-5.

Belgorosky A, Rivarola MA. Progressive increase in non-SHBG-bound testosterone and estradiol from infancy to late prepuberty in girls. J Clin Endocrinol Metab 1988 Aug;67(2):234-7.

Christiansen KH. Serum and saliva sex hormone levels in Kung San men. Am J Phys Anthropol 1991;86(1):37-44.

Cooke RR, McIntosh JE, McIntosh RP. Circadian variation in serum free and non-SHBG-bound testosterone in normal men: measurements and simulation using a mass action model. Clin Endocrinol (Oxf) 1993 Aug;39(2):163-71.

Corradi G, Szathmari M . Serum and salivary testosterone levels in erectile dysfunction. Orv Hetil 1998 Aug 23;139(34):2021-24.

Davison SL, R Bell R, Donath S, Montalto JG , Davis SR. androgen levels in adult females: changes with age. Journal of Clinical Endocrinology & Metabolism. First published April 12, 2005.

Fahrner CL, Hackney AC. Effects of endurance exercise on free testosterone concentration and the binding affinity of sex hormone binding globulin (SHBG). Int J Sports Med 1998 Jan;19(1):12-25.

Govier FE, McClure RD, Kramer-Levien D. Endocrine screening for sexual dysfunction using free testosterone determinations. J Urol. 1996 Aug;156(2 Pt 1):405-08.

Hardy KJ, Seckl JR. Endocrine assessment of impotence-pitfalls of measuring serum testosterone without sex-hormone-binding globulin. Postgraduate Med Journal. 1994 Nov;70(829):836-7.

Khan-Dawood FS, Choe JK, Dawood MY. Salivary and plasma bound and "free" testosterone in men and women. Am J Obstet Gynecol 1984 Feb 15;148(4):441-5.

Kuhn JM, et al. Studies on the treatment of idiopathic gynaecomastia with percutaneous DHT or dihydrotestosterone. Clin Endocrinol (Oxf) 1983 Oct;19(4):513-20.

Michael A, Jenaway A, Paykel ES, Herbert J. Altered salivary dehydroepi androsterone levels in major depression in adults. Biol Psychiatry 2000 Nov 15;48(10):989-95.

Mohr B, Guay AT, O'Donnell AB, McKinlay JB, Morley JE, et al. Normal, bound and nonbound testosterone levels in normally ageing men: results from the Massachusetts Male Ageing Study. Clinical Endocrinology (2005) 62, 64-73.

Longitudinal changes in testosterone, luteinizing hormone and follicle-stimulating hormone in healthy men. Metabolism 1997 Apr;46(4):410-13.

Nawata H, Kato K, Ibayashi H. Age-dependent change of serum 5alpha-dihydrotestosterone and its relation to testosterone in man. Endocrinology J. 1977 Feb;24(1):41-5.

Pirke KM, Doerr P. Plasma dihydrotestosterone in normal adult males and its relation to testosterone. Acta Endocrinol (Copenh) 1975 Jun;79(2):357-65.

Rilling JK, et al. Ratios of plasma and salivary testosterone throughout puberty: production versus bioavailability. Steroids 1996 Jun;61(6):374-8.

Tilakaratne A, Soory M. androgen metabolism in response to oestradiol-17beta and progesterone in human gingival fibroblasts (HGF) in culture. J Clin Periodontol 1999 Nov;26(11):723-31.

Vermeulen A, Verdonck L, Kaufman JM. A critical evaluation of simple methods for the estimation of free testosterone in serum. J Clin Endocrinol Metab 1999 Oct;84(10):3666-72 Comment in: J Clin Endocrinol Metab. 2001 Jun;86(6):2903.

Melatonin, Prolactin and Biological Rhythms

Anderson RA, Lincoln GA, Wu FC. Melatonin potentiates testosterone-induced suppression of luteinizing hormone secretion in normal men. Hum Reprod 1993 Nov;8(11):1819-22.

Cagnacci A. Melatonin in relation to physiology in adult humans. Pineal Res 1996 Nov;21(4):200-13.

Czeisler C, Duffy J, Shanahan T, et al. Stability, precision and near-24-hour period of the human circadian pacemaker. Science. 1999;284:2177-81.

Dawson D, van den Heuvel CJ, Integrating the actions of melatonin on human physiology. Ann Med 1998 Feb;30(1):95-102.

Drobnik J, Dabrowski R. Pinealectomy-induced elevation of collagen content in the intact skin is suppressed by melatonin application. Cytobios 1999;100(393):49-55.

Fruchtman S, Jackson L, Borski R. Insulin-like growth factor I disparately regulates prolactin and growth hormone synthesis and secretion: studies using the teleost pituitary model. Endocrinology. 2000 Aug;141(8):2886-94.

Gilad E, Matzkin H, Zisapel N. Interplay between sex steroids and melatonin in regulation of human benign prostate epithelial cell growth. Clin Endocrinol Metab 1997 Aug;82(8):2535-41

Hanse L, Bedel M. Psychotic Episode After Melatonin. Annals of Pharmacology. 1977;31:1408.

Kostoglou-Athanassiou I, Treacher DF, Wheeler MJ, Forsling ML. Bright light exposure and pituitary hormone secretion. Clin Endocrinol (Oxf) 1998 Jan;48(1):73-9

Kumar V. Melatonin: a master hormone and a candidate for universal panacea. Indian J Exp Biol 1996 May;34(5):391-402.

Nowak JZ, Zawilska JB. Melatonin and its physiological and therapeutic properties. Pharm World Sci 1998 Feb;20(1):18-27.

Ohashi Y, et al. Differential pattern of the circadian rhythm of serum melatonin in young and elderly healthy subjects. Biol Signals 1997 Jul-Dec;6(4-6):301-03.

Okatani Y, Morioka N, Wakatsuki A . Changes in nocturnal melatonin secretion in perimenopausal women: correlation with endogenous estrogen concentrations. J Pineal Res 2000 Mar;28(2):111-8.

Petterborg LJ, Thalen BE, Kjellman BF, Wetterberg L. Effect of melatonin replacement on serum hormone rhythms in a patient lacking endogenous melatonin. Brain Res Bull 1991 Aug;27(2):181-5.

Pevet P. Melatonin and biological rhythms. Biol Signals Recept 2000 May-Aug;9(3-4):203-12.

Rubin RT, Pol and RE, Tower BB. Prolactin-related testosterone secretion in normal adult men. Clin Endocrinol Metab 1976 Jan;42(1):112-16.

Van Cauter E, Plat L, Leproult R, Copinschi G. Alterations of circadian rhythmicity and sleep in aging: endocrine consequences. Horm Res. 1998;49:147-152.

Webley GE, Bohle A, Leidenberger FA. Positive relationship between the nocturnal concentrations of melatonin and prolactin and a stimulation of prolactin after melatonin administration in young men. J Pineal Res 1988;5(1):19-33.

Weitzman ED, et al. Studies of the 24 hour rhythm of melatonin in man. Neural Transm Suppl 1978;(13):325-33.

Winters SJ. Diurnal rhythm of testosterone and luteinizing hormone in hypogonadal men. J Androl 1991 May-Jun;12(3):185-90.

Zhdanova IV, Wurtman RJ, et al. Melatonin treatment for age-related insomnia. J Clin Endocrinol Metab 2001 Oct;86(10):4727-30.

Miscellaneous

Abrams, D. Use of androgens in Patients Who Have HIV/AIDS: What We Know About the Effect of androgens on Wasting and Lipodystrophy The AIDS Reader 2001; 11(3):149-156.

Allen NE, Appleby PN, Davey GK, Key TJ. Soymilk intake in relation to serum sex hormone levels in British men. Nutr Cancer. 2001;41(1-2):41-6.

Bertone-Johnson ER. Calcium and Vitamin D may Prevent PMS. Archives of Internal Medicine. June13, 2005;165(11);1246-52.

Bowles JT. Sex, kings and serial killers and other group-selected human traits. Med Hypotheses. 2000 Jun;54(6):864-94. JeffBo@aol.com

Christiansen D, Weight Matters, Even in the Womb. Science News, Dec 9, 2000;158:382-83.

Dougherty RH, et al. Effect of aromatase inhibition on lipids and inflammatory markers of cardiovascular disease in elderly men with low testosterone levels. Clinical Endocrinol.2005 Feb; 62(2):228-35.

Dzugan SA, Arnold Smith R. Hypercholesterolemia treatment: a new hypothesis or just an accident? Med Hypotheses 2002 Nov;59(6):751-6.

el-Awady MK, Salam MA, Gad YZ, el-Saban J. Dihydrotestosterone regulates plasma sex-hormone-binding globulin in prepubertal males: Clin Endocrinol (Oxf) 1989 Mar;30(3):279-84.

Fink G, Sumner B, Rosie R, Wilson H, McQueen J. androgen actions on central serotonin neurotransmission: relevance for mood, mental state and memory. Behav Brain Res 1999 Nov 1;105(1):53-68.

Guay AT, Bansal S, Hodge MB. Possible hypothalamic impotence. Male counterpart to hypothalamic amenorrhea? Urology 1991 Oct;38(4):317-22.

Guay, AT. Director, Center for Sexual Function/Endocrinology; Lahey Clinic Northshore, One Essex Center Drive, Peabody, MA. 01960. Personal Communication. November 14, 2003. Andre.T.Guay@lahey.org

*Leder BZ, Finkelstein JS. Effect of aromatase inhibition on bone metabolism in elderly hypogonadal men. Osteoporosis Int. 2005; (Epub ahead of print) bzleder@partnrs.org

Hayashi T, et al. Dehydroepiandrosterone Retards Atherosclerosis Formation Through Its Conversion to Estrogen: The Possible Role of Nitric Oxide. Arterioscler Thromb Vasc Biol 2000 Mar;20(3):782-792.

*Makhsida N, et al. Hypogonadism and Metabolic Syndrome Implications for Testosterone Therapy. J of Urology 2005 Sep;174:827-834.

Mokdad AH, Marks JS, Stroup, DF , Gerberding JL. Actual Causes of Death in the United States, 2000. JAMA, Mar10,2004;(291)10:1238-45.

Ness, J, Sherman, F T, Pan CX. Alternative Medicine: What the data say about common herbal therapies. Geriatrics 1999;54 (10) 33-43.

Seeman M. Psychopathology in women and men: focus on female hormones. Am J Psychiatry, 1997; Dec.154:12.

Seppa N. Cetenarian Advantage. Science News 2003, October 18, 164; 243.

Shively CA, et al. Soy and social stress affect serotonin neurotransmission in primates. Pharmacogenomics J. 2003;3(2):114-21.

Strain GW, et al. Effect of massive weight loss on hypothalamic-pituitary-gonadal function in obese men. J Clin Endocrinol Metab 1988 May;66(5):1019-23.

Trichopoulou A, Costacou T, Bamia C, Trichopoulos D. Adherence to a Mediterranean diet and survival in a Greek population. NEJM 2003 Jun 26;348(26):2595-96.

Weiner, Leslie. Vegetarianism and health. Special Report. *Nutrition Research Newsletter* 1988; 8:123-27.

Werbach, Melvyn R. Nutritional Therapy: An Important Component of Integrative Medicine. 2004 July/Aug; 10(4): 12-13.

van de Weijer Peter HM, Barensten Ronald. Isoflavones from red clover (Promensil®) significantly reduce menopausal hot flush symptoms compared with placebo. Maturitas 2002;42:187-93.

van Niekerk JK, Huppert FA, Herbert J. Salivary cortisol and DHEA: association with measures of cognition and well-being in normal older men and effects of three months of DHEA supplementation. Psychoneuroendocrinology 2001 Aug;26(6):591-612.

*Weil Andrew. NUTRITION AND HEALTH. Explore January 2005;1(1):65-66.

Vojta CL, Fraga PD, Forciea MA, Lavizzo-Mourey R. anti-aging Therapy: An Overview. Hospital Practice. June15, 2001;43-49.

Older Men, Memory and Testosterone

Arlt W, et al. Biotransformation of oral dehydroepi androsterone in elderly men: significant increase in circulating estrogens. Clinical Journal of Endocrinology and Metabolism 1999 Jun;84(6):2170-76.

Bain J. andropause: Testosterone replacement therapy for aging men. Can Fam Physician 2001 Jan;47:91-97.

Bhasin S, Buckwater JG. Testosterone supplementation in older men-A rational idea whose time has not yet come. J. Androl. 2001;22:718-31.

Bowles J, The evolution of aging: A new approach to an old problem of biology. Med Hyptheses 1998; 51:179-221.

Bowen RL, et al. Elevated luteinizing hormone expression localizes with neurons vulnerable to Alzheimer's disease pathology. J Neuroscience Research 2002 Nov 1;70(3):514-18.

Cherrier MM, et al. Testosterone supplementation improves spatial and verbal memory in healthy older men. Neurology 2001 Jul 10;57(1):80-88.

Cherrier MM, et al. The role of aromatization in testosterone supplementation: effects on cognition in older men. Neurology 2005 Jan;64(2):2990-96.

Gouchie C, Kimura D. The relationship between testosterone levels and cognitive ability patterns. Psychoneuroendocrinology 1991;16(4):323-34.

Heaton JP, Morales A. andropause a multisystem disease. Can J Urol 2001 Apr;8(2):1213-22.

Friedrich MJ. Biological Secrets of Exceptional Old Age: Centenarian Study Seeks Insight into Aging Well. JAMA 11/2002;288:18:2247.

Gambert S. andropause and the Aging Male. Clinical Geriatrics 2003 Jan;11(1):12-13.

Ly LP, et al. A double-blind, placebo-controlled, randomized clinical trial of transdermal dihydrotestosterone gel on muscular strength, mobility and quality of life in older men with partial androgen deficiency. J Clin Endocrinol Metab 2001 Sep;86(9):4078-88.

Nankin HR, Calkins JH. Decreased bioavailable testosterone in aging normal and impotent men. J Clin Endocrinol Metab 1986 Dec;63(6):1418-20.

Morley JE, et al. Longitudinal changes in testosterone, luteinizing hormone and follicle-stimulating hormone in healthy older men. Metabolism 1997 Apr;46(4):410-13.

Morley JE. andropause, testosterone therapy and quality of life in aging men. Cleve Clin J Med 2000 Dec;67(12):880-82.

Morley JE Testosterone replacement in older men and women. J Gend Specif Med 2001;4(2):49-53.

Plymate SR, Tenover JS, Bremner WJ. Circadian variation in testosterone, sex hormone-binding globulin and calculated non-sex hormone-binding globulin bound testosterone in healthy young and elderly men. J Androl 1989 Sep-Oct;10(5):366-71.

Swartz, C. Low Serum Testosterone: a Cardiovascular Risk in Elderly Men. Geriatric Medicine Today. 1988, Dec; 7:12.

Tenover JS, Matsumoto AM, Plymate SR, Bremner WJ. The effects of aging in normal men on bioavailable testosterone and luteinizing hormone secretion: response to clomiphene citrate. J Clin Endocrinol Metab 1987 Dec;65(6):1118-26.

Urban RJ, et al. Testosterone administration to elderly men increases skeletal muscle strength and protein synthesis. Am J Physiol 1995 Nov;269(5 Pt 1):E820-26.

Veldhuis JD, Iranmanesh A, Mulligan T, Pincus SM. Disruption of the young-adult synchrony between luteinizing hormone release and oscillations in follicle-stimulating hormone, prolactin and nocturnal penile tumescence (NPT) in healthy older men. J Clin Endocrinol Metab. 1999 Oct;84(10):3498-505.

Winters SJ, Sherins RJ, Troen P. The gonadotropin-suppressive activity of androgen is increased in elderly men. Metabolism 1984 Nov;33(11):1052-59.

Oxytocin, the Loving Hormone

Argiolas A, Melis MR, Murgia S, Schioth HB. ACTH- and alpha-MSH-induced grooming, stretching, yawning and penile erection in male rats: site of action in the brain and role of melanocortin receptors. Brain Res Bull. 2000 Mar 15;51(5):425-31. argiolas@unica.it

Anderson-Hunt M, Dennerstein L. Increased female sexual response after oxytocin. BMJ 1994;309:929.

Anderson-Hunt M, Dennerstein L. Oxytocin and female sexuality. Gynecol Obstet Invest 1995;40(4):217-21.

Arletti R, Benelli A, Bertolini A. Oxytocin involvement in male and female sexual behavior. Ann NY Acad Sci 1992;652:180-93.

Blaicher W, et al. The role of oxytocin in relation to female sexual arousal.

Gynecol Obstet Invest 1999;47(2):125-6.

Cantor JM, Binik YM, Pfaus JG. Chronic fluoxetine inhibits sexual behavior in the male rat: reversal with oxytocin. Psychopharmacology (Berl) 1999 Jun;144(4):355-62.

Carter SC, et al. Oxytocin and social bonding. Ann NY Acad Sci 1992;652:204-11.

Carmichael MS, Warburton VL, Dixen J, Davidson JM. Relationships among cardiovascular, muscular and oxytocin responses during human sexual activity. Arch Sex Behav 1994 Feb;23(1):59-79.

Gimpl G, Fahrenholz F. The oxytocin receptor system: structure, function and regulation. Physiological Reviews 2001 Apr;81(2):629-83.

Insel TR. Post-partum increases in brain oxytocin binding. Neuroendocrinology 1986;44:515-18.

Ivell R, et al. Oxytocin and male reproductive function. Adv Exp Med Biol 1997;424:253-64.

Kendrick KM, Keverne EB, Baldwin BA. Intracerebroventricular oxytocin stimulates maternal behaviour in the sheep. Neuroendocrinology 1987;46:56-61.

Kuhn JM, et al. Effects of 10 days administration of percutaneous dihydrotestosterone on the pituitary-testicular axis in normal men. Clin Endocrinol Metab 1984 Feb;58(2):231-5.

McCarthy MM. Estrogen modulation of oxytocin and its relation to behavior. Adv Exp Med Biol 1995;395:235-45.

Meuleman EJ, et al. A neuropeptide in human semen: oxytocin. Arch Androl 1998 Jul-Aug;41(1):17-22.

Molinoff PB,et al. PT-141: a melanocortin agonist for the treatment of sexual dysfunction. Ann N Y Acad Sci. 2003 Jun;994:96-102.

Murphy MR, et al. Changes in oxytocin and vasopressin secretion during sexual activity in men. Journal of Clinical Endocrinology & Metabolism 1987 Oct;65(4):738-41.

Murphy MR, Checkley SA, Seckl JR, Lightman SL. Naloxone inhibits oxytocin release at orgasm in man. J Clin Endocrinol Metab 1990 Oct;71(4):1056-58.

Nicholson HD, Jenkin L. Oxytocin and prostatic function. Prostate 1999 Sept 1;40(4):211-17.

Nicholson HD, Pickering BT. Oxytocin, a male intragonadal hormone. Regul Pept 1993 Apr 29;45(1-2):253-56.

Ogawa S, Kudo S, Kitsunai Y, Fukuchi S. Increase in oxytocin secretion at ejaculation in male. Clin Endocrinol (Oxf) 1980 Jul;13(1):95-97.

Pedersen CA, Ascher JA, Monroe YL, Prange AJ. Oxytocin induces maternal behavior in virgin female rats. Science 1982;216:649-84.

Sabatier N, et al. Oxytocin released from magnocellular dendrites: a potential modulator of alpha-melanocyte-stimulating hormone behavioral actions? Ann N Y Acad Sci. 2003 Jun;994:218-24.

Voisey J, Carroll L, van Daal A. Melanocortins and their receptors and antagonists. Curr Drug Targets. 2003 Oct;4(7):586-97.

Watson ED, Nikolakopoulos E, Gilbert C, Goode J. Oxytocin in the semen and gonads of the stallion. Theriogenology 1999 Mar;51(4):855-65.

Young LJ, Lim MM, Gingrich B, Insel TR. Cellular mechanisms of social attachment. Hormonal Behavior 2001 Sep;40(2):133-38.

Progesterone, Sleep and Testosterone

Baulieu EE, Schumacher M. Progesterone as a neuroactive neurosteroid, with special reference to the effect of progesterone on myelination. Human Reproduction 2000 Jun;15 (1):1-13.

Brady BM Anderson RA, Kinniburgh D, Baird DT. Demonstration of progesterone receptor-mediated gonadotrophin suppression in the human male. Clin Endocrinol (Oxf) 2003 Apr;58(4):506-12.

Barfield RJ. Glaser JH. Rubin BS. Etgen AM. Behavioral effects of progestin in the brain. [Review] Psychoneuroendocrinology.1984; 9(3):217-31.

Brown DV, Amann RP. Inhibition of testosterone metabolism in cultured rat epididymal principal cells by dihydrotestosterone and progesterone. Biol Reproduction 1984 Feb;30(1):67-73.

Cabeza M, et al. Anti androgenic effect of new synthetic steroids. Proc West Pharmacol Soc. 2000;43:31-32.

Cabeza M, et al. Evaluation of new pregnane derivatives as 5alpha-reductase inhibitor. Chem Pharm Bull (Tokyo). 2001 May;49(5):525-30.

Carmody BJ, et al. Progesterone inhibits human infragenicular arterial smooth muscle cell proliferation induced by high glucose and insulin concentrations. J Vasc Surg 2002 Oct;36(4):833-38.

Cistulli PA, Grunstein RR, Sullivan CE. Effect of testosterone administration on upper airway collapsibility during sleep. Am Journal Respir Crit Care Med 1994 Feb;149(2 Pt 1):530-32.

Dewis P, Newman M Anderson DC. The effect of endogenous progesterone on serum levels of 5 alpha-reduced androgens in hirsute women. Clin Endocrinol (Oxf) 1984 Oct;21(4):383-92.

Finn MM, et al. The frequency of salivary progesterone sampling and the diagnosis of luteal phase insufficiency. Gynecol Endocrinol 1992 Jun;6(2):127-34.

Fleischmann A. Etgen AM. Makman MH. Estradiol plus progesterone promote glutamate-induced release of gamma-aminobutyric acid from preoptic area synaptosomes. Neuropharmacology. 1992;31(8):799-807.

Fortune JE, Vincent SE. Progesterone inhibits the induction of aromatase activity in rat granulosa cells in vitro. Biol Reprod 1983 Jun;28(5):1078-89.

Genazzani AR,et al. Effects of sex steroid hormones on the neuroendocrine system. Eur J Contracept Reprod Health Care 1997 Mar;2(1):63-9.

Genazzani AR, et al. Progesterone, progestagens and the central nervous system. Hum Reprod 2000 Jun;15 Suppl 1:14-27.

Grunstein RR, et al. Neuroendocrine dysfunction in sleep apnea: reversal by continuous positive airways pressure therapy. J Clin Endocrinol Metab 1989 Feb;68(2):352-58.

Kapsimalis F, Kryger MH. Gender and obstructive sleep apnea syndrome, part 2: mechanisms. Sleep 2002 Aug 1;25(5):499-506.

Koenig HL, et al. Progesterone synthesis and myelin formation by Schwan cells. Science 1995 Jun 9;268(5216):1500-3.

Koenig HL, Gong WH, Pelissier P. Role of progesterone in peripheral nerve repair. Rev Reprod 2000 Sep;5(3):189-99.

Kouchiyama S, et al. Prediction of the degree of nocturnal oxygen desaturation in sleep apnea syndrome by estimating the testosterone level. Nihon Kyobu Shikkan Gakkai Zasshi 1989 Aug;27(8):941-5.

Leb CR, Hu FY, Murphy BE. Metabolism of progesterone by human lymphocytes: production of neuroactive steroids. J Clin Endocrinol Metab 1997 Dec;82(12):4064-48.

Matsumoto AM, et al. Testosterone replacement in hypogonadal men: effects on obstructive sleep apnoea, respiratory drives and sleep. Clin Endocrinol (Oxf) 1985 Jun;22(6):713-21.

Mauvais-Jarvis P, Kuttenn F, Wright F. Progesterone administered by percutaneous route: an anti androgen locally useful]. Annals of Endocrinology (Paris) 1975 Mar-Apr;36(2):55-62.

Manber R, Kuo TF, Cataldo N, Colrain IM. The effects of hormone replacement therapy on sleep-disordered breathing in postmenopausal women: a pilot study. Sleep

Meulenberg PM, Hofman JA. Salivary progesterone excellently reflects free and total progesterone in plasma during pregnancy. Chem 1989 Jan;35(1):168-72.

Mohr PE, Wang DY, Gregory WM, Richards MA, Fentiman IS. Serum progesterone and prognosis in operable breast cancer. Br J Cancer 1996 Jun;73(12):1552-5.

Muneyyirci-Delale O, et al. Serum ionized magnesium and calcium and sex hormones in healthy young men: importance of serum progesterone level. Fertil Steril 1999 Nov;72(5):817-22.

Netzer NC, Eliasson AH, Strohl KP. Women with sleep apnea have lower levels of sex hormones. Sleep Breath 2003 Mar;7(1):25-30.

Phelps SM, Lydon JP, O'Malley BW, Crews D. Regulation of Male Sexual Behavior by Progesterone Receptor, Sexual Experience and androgen. Hormones and Behavior 1998; 34, 294-302.

Reid RL Progestins in hormone replacement therapy: Impact on endometrial and breast cancer. J. SOCGC.2000 Sep;22(9):677-681.

Saaresranta T, Polo O. Hormones and breathing. Chest 2002 Dec;122(6):2165-82

Santamaria JD, Prior JC, Fleetham JA. Reversible reproductive dysfunction in men with obstructive sleep apnoea. Clin Endocrinol (Oxf) 1988 May;28(5):461-70.

Schairer C. Progesterone receptors - animal models and cell signalling in breast cancer: Implications for breast cancer of inclusion of progestins in hormone replacement therapies. Breast Cancer Res 2002;4(6):244-48.

Schiavi RC, White D, Mandeli J. Pituitary-gonadal function during sleep in healthy aging men. Psychoneuroendocrinology 1992 Nov;17(6):599-609.

Shahar E, et al. Hormone Replacement Therapy and Sleep-disordered Breathing. Am J Respir Crit Care Med 2003 May 1;167(9):1186-92.

Sherwin BB. The impact of different doses of estrogen and progestin on mood and sexual behavior in postmenopausal women. J Clin Endocrinol Metab. 1991 Feb;72(2):336-43.

Steiner M, Dunn E, Born L. Hormones and mood: from menarche to menopause and beyond. J Affect Disord 2003 Mar;74(1):67-83.

Tilakaratne A, Soory M. androgen metabolism in response to oestradiol-17beta and progesterone in human gingival fibroblasts (HGF) in culture. J Clin Periodontol 1999 Nov;26(11):723-31.

White DP, et al. Influence of testosterone on ventilation and chemosensitivity in male subjects. J Appl Physiol 1985 Nov;59(5):1452-57.

Prostate and Testosterone

Alavanja MC, et al. Use of agricultural pesticides and prostate cancer risk in the Agricultural Health Study cohort. Am J Epidemiol. 2003 May 1;157(9):800-14.

Barrett-Connor E, et al. A prospective, population-based study of androstenedione, estrogens and prostatic cancer. Cancer Res 1990 Jan 1;50(1):169-73.

Bartsch G, Rittmaster RS, Klocker H. Dihydrotestosterone and the concept of 5alpha-reductase inhibition in human benign prostatic hyperplasia. Eur Urol 2000 Apr;37(4):367-80

Berthaut I, et al. Pharmacological and molecular evidence for the expression of the two steroid 5 alpha-reductase isozymes in normal and hyperplastic human prostatic cells in culture. Prostate 1997 Aug 1;32(3):155-63.

Bonkhoff H, Stein U, Aumuller G, Remberger K. Differential expression of 5 alpha-reductase isoenzymes in the human prostate and prostatic carcinomas. Prostate 1996 Oct;29(4):261-7

Carroll K et al. A link Between Diet and Cancer of the Prostate. Progressive Biochemical Pharmacology 1975; 10:308.

Chan JM, Stampfer MJ, et al. Plasma insulin-like growth factor I and prostate cancer risk: a prospective study. Science 1998;279:563-566.

Guay AT, Perez JB, Fitaihi WA, Vereb M. Testosterone treatment in hypogonadal men: prostate-specific antigen level and risk of prostate cancer. Endocr Pract. 2000 Mar-Apr;6(2):132-8.

Gustafsson O, et al. Dihydrotestosterone and testosterone levels in men screened for prostate cancer: a study of a randomized population. Br J Urol 1996 Mar;77(3):433-40.

Habib FK, et al. The localization and expression of 5 alpha-reductase types I and II mRNAs in human hyperplastic prostate and in prostate primary cultures. J Endocrinol. 1998 Mar;156(3):509-17.

Habib FK, Ross M, Bayne CW. Factors controlling the expression of 5alpha-reductase in human prostate: A possible new approach for the treatment of prostate cancer. Eur Urol 1999;35(5-6):439-42.

Hajjar RR. et al. Benign Prostatic Hypertropy. J Clin Endo Metab 1997;82:3793-96.

Heikkila R, et al. Serum testosterone and sex hormone-binding globulin concentrations and the risk of prostate carcinoma: a longitudinal study. Cancer 1999 Jul 15;86(2):312-5.

Iehle C, et al. Differences in steroid 5alpha-reductase iso-enzymes expression between normal and pathological human prostate tissue. J Steroid Biochem Mol Biol. 1999 Mar;68(5-6):189-95.

Jiang Q, Wong J, Ames BN Gamma-tocopherol induces apoptosis in androgen-responsive LNCaP prostate cancer cells via caspase-dependent and independent mechanisms. Ann N Y Acad Sci, 2004 Dec; 1031:399-4.

Krieg M, Schlenker A, Voigt KD. Inhibition of androgen metabolism in stroma and epithelium of the human benign prostatic hyperplasia by progesterone, estrone and estradiol. Prostate 1985;6(3):233-40.

Kyprianou N, Isaacs JT. Quantal relationship between prostatic dihydrotestosterone and prostatic cell content: critical threshold concept. Prostate 1987;11(1):41-50.

Mahendroo MS, Russell DW. Male and female isoenzymes of steroid 5alpha-reductase. Rev Reprod 1999 Sep;4(3):179-83.

McConnell J. et al. Medical Therapy of Prostatic Symptoms. Program Abstracts of the American Urological Association 2002. Annual Meeting (Abstract 1042, updated)

Meikle AW, Smith JA, Stringham JD. Estradiol and testosterone metabolism and production in men with prostatic cancer. J Steroid Biochem 1989 Jul;33(1):19-24.

Meikle AW, Smith JA, Stringham JD. Production, clearance and metabolism of testosterone in men with prostatic cancer. Prostate 1987;10(1):25-31.

Melcangi RC, et al. The 5alpha-reductase in the central nervous system: expression and modes of control. J Steroid Biochem Mol Biol 1998 Apr;65(1-6):295-9.

Mills PK, Yang R. Prostate cancer risk in California farm workers. J Occup Environ Med. 2003 Mar;45(3):249-58.

Morgentaler A. Is low serum free testosterone a marker for high grade prostate cancer? J Urol 2000 Mar;163(3):824-7.

Prehn RT. On the prevention and therapy of prostate cancer by androgen administration. Cancer Res 1999 Sep 1;59(17):4161-64.

Randall VA. Role of 5 alpha-reductase in health and disease. Baillieres Clin Endocrinol Metab 1994 Apr;8(2):405-31.

Radical Prostates. Female hormones may play a pivotal role in a distinctly male epidemic. Science News. Feb 22,1997; (151) 126-127.

Rennie PS, et al. Kinetic analysis of 5 alpha-reductase isoenzymes in benign prostatic hyperplasia (BPH). J Steroid Biochem 1983 Jul;19(1A):169-73.

Rimler A, Matzkin H, Zisapel N. Cross talk between melatonin and TGF-beta-1 in human benign prostate epithelial cells. J Clin Endocrinol Metab 2001;86:694-699.

Sciarra F. Effects of sex steroids and Epidermal Growth Factor (EGF) in benign prostatic hyperplasia (BPH). Ann N Y Acad Sci 1995;761: 66-78.

Shibata Y, et al. Changes in the endocrine environment of the human prostate transition zone with aging: simultaneous quantitative analysis of prostatic sex steroids and comparison with human prostatic histological composition. Prostate 2000 Jan;42(1):45-55.

Steers WD. 5alpha-reductase activity in the prostate. Urology. 2001

Dec;58(6 Suppl 1):17-24; discussion 24.

Travis J. Do Arctic Diets protect prostates? Science News 2003, Oct;164: 253.

Thompson I. et al. The Influence of Finasteride on the development of Prostate Cancer. New England Journal of Medicine 2003; 349:213.

Weisser H, Krieg M. In vitro inhibition of androstenedione 5alpha-reduction by finasteride in epithelium and stroma of human benign prostatic hyperplasia. J Steroid Biochem Mol Biol. 1998 Oct;67(1):49-55.

Weisser H, Krieg M. Benign prostatic hyperplasia-the outcome of age-induced alteration of androgen-estrogen balance? Urologe A 1997 Jan;36(1):3-9.

Winters SJ, et al. Testosterone, sex hormone-binding globulin and body composition in young adult African American and Caucasian men. Metabolism.2001 Oct;50(10):1242-7.

Sexual Function and Testosterone

Adaikan PG, Srilatha B. Oestrogen-mediated hormonal imbalance precipitates erectile dysfunction. Int J Impot Res 2003 Feb;15(1):38-43.

Alexander GM,et al. Mood and response to auditory sexual stimuli. Horm Behav 1997 Apr;31(2):110-19.

Anderson RA, Bancroft J, Wu FC. The effects of exogenous testosterone on sexuality and mood of normal men. J Clin Endocrinol Metab 1992 Dec;75(6):1503-7.

Arver S, et al. Improvement of sexual function in testosterone deficient men treated for 1 year with a permeation enhanced testosterone transdermal system. J Urol 1996 May;155(5):1604-06.

Bagatell CJ, Heiman JR, Rivier JE, Bremner WJ. Effects of endogenous testosterone and estradiol on sexual behavior in normal young men. J Clin Endocrinol Metab 1994 Mar;78(3):711-6 in: J Clin Endocrinol Metab 1994 Jun;78(6):1520.

Bohlen JG, Held JP, Sanderson MO. The male orgasm: pelvic contractions measured by anal probe. Arch Sex Behav 1980 Dec;9(6):503-21.

Brown WA, Monti PM, Corriveau DP. Serum testosterone and sexual activity and interest in men. Arch Sex Behav 1978 Mar;7(2):97-103.

Carani C, et al. Effects of androgen treatment in impotent men with normal and low levels of free testosterone. Arch Sex Behav 1990 Jun;19(3):223-34.

Carani C, Granata AR, Fustini MF, Marrama P. Prolactin and testosterone: their role in male sexual function. Int J Androl 1996 Feb;19(1):48-54.

Carmichael MS, Warburton VL, Dixen J, Davidson JM. Relationships among cardiovascular, muscular and oxytocin responses during human sexual activity. Arch Sex Behav 1994 Feb;23(1):59-79.

Christiansen K, Knussmann R. Sex hormones and cognitive functioning in men. Neuropsychobiology 1987;18(1):27-36.

Clopper RR, et al. Psychosexual behavior in hypopituitary men: a controlled comparison of gonadotropin and testosterone replacement. Psychoneuroendocrinology 1993;18(2):149-61.

Davidson JM, Camargo CA, Smith ER. Effects of androgen on sexual behavior in hypogonadal men. Metab 1979 Jun;48(6):955-8

Exton MS, et al. Cardiovascular and endocrine alterations after masturbation-induced orgasm in women. Psychosom Med 1999 May-Jun;61(3):280-91.

Exton NG, et al. Neuroendocrine response to film-induced sexual arousal in men and women. Psychoneuroendocrinology 2000 Feb;25(2):187-99.

Fabbri A, Caprio M, Aversa A. Pathology of erection. J Endocrinol Invest. 2003;26(3 Suppl):87-90.

Gooren LJ. androgen levels and sex functions in testosterone-treated hypogonadal men. Arch Sex Behav 1987 Dec;16(6):463-73.

Jannini EA, et al. Lack of sexual activity from erectile dysfunction is associated with a reversible reduction in serum testosterone. Int J Androl 1999 Dec;22(6):385-92

Keefe DL. Sex hormones and neural mechanisms. Arch Sex Behavior 2002 Oct;31(5):401-3.

Knussmann R, Christiansen K, Couwenbergs C. Relations between sex hormone levels and sexual behavior in men. Arch Sex Behav 1986 Oct;15(5):429-45.

Kruger T, et al. Neuroendocrine and cardiovascular response to sexual arousal and orgasm in men. Psychoneuroendocrinology 1998 May;23(4):401-11.

Laumann EO, Paik A, Rosen RC. Sexual dysfunction in the United States: prevalence and predictors. JAMA 1999 Feb 10;281(6):537-44.

Mantzoros CS, Georgiadis EI, Trichopoulos D. Contribution of dihydrotestosterone to male sexual behaviour. BMJ 1995; 310, 6990:1289-91.

Meston CM, Frohlich PF. The Neurobiology of Sexual Function Arch Gen Psychiatry. 2000;57:1012-1030.

Schwartz MF, Kolodny RC, Masters WH. Plasma testosterone levels of sexually functional and dysfunctional men. Arch Sex Behav 1980 Oct;9(5):355-66.

Nicolosi A, et al. Epidemiology of erectile dysfunction in four countries: cross national study of the prevalence and correlates of erectile dysfunction. Urology 2003 Jan;61(1):201-6.

Nusbaum MR. Erectile dysfunction: prevalence, etiology and major risk factors. J Am Osteopath Assoc 2002 Dec;102(12 Suppl 4):S1-6.

Rakic Z, Starcevic V, Starcevic VP, Marinkovic J . Testosterone treatment in men with erectile disorder and low levels of total testosterone in serum. Arch Sex Behav 1997 Oct;26(5):495-504.

Riley A; Riley E. Controlled studies on women presenting with sexual drive disorder: I. Endocrine status. J Sex Marital Ther 2000 Jul;26(3):269-283.

Schwartz MF, Kolodny RC, Masters WH. Plasma testosterone levels of sexually functional and dysfunctional men. Arch Sex Behav 1980 Oct;9(5):355-66.

Turner BB. Influence of gonadal steroids on brain corticosteroid receptors: a mini review. Neurochem Res. 1997 Nov;22(11):1375-85.

Sperm Counts and Testosterone

Auger J, Kunstmann JM, Cazyglik F, Jouannet P. Decline in semen quality among fertile men in Paris during the past 20 years. N Engl J Med 1995; 332:281.

Hudson RW, et al. Seminal plasma testosterone and dihydrotestosterone levels in men with varicoceles. Int J Androl 1983 Apr;6(2):135-42.

Irvine, S, et al. Evidence of deteriorating semen quality in the United Kingdom: Birth cohort study in 577 men in Scotland over 11 years. Br Med J 1996; 312:467.

Le Lannou D, et al. Testosterone and 5 alpha-dihydrotestosterone concentrations in human seminal plasma. Int J Androl 1980 Oct;3(5):502-6.

Murray TJ, et al. Endocrine disrupting chemicals: Effects on human male reproductive health. Early Pregnancy 2001 Apr;5(2):80-112.

Pavlovich CP, Goldstein M. Hormonal Regulation of Spermatogenesis J Urol 2001;165:837-841.

Sharpe RM, Skakkebaek NE. Are oestrogens involved in falling sperm counts and disorders of the male reproductive tract? Lancet 1993;431:1392-95.

Yamamoto M, et al. In-vitro contractility of human seminiferous tubules in response to testosterone, dihydrotestosterone and estradiol. Urol Res 1989;17(4):265-8.

Transdermal Testosterones

Arver S et al, Improvement of sexual function in testosterone deficient men treated for 1 year with a permeation enhanced testosterone transdermal system, J Urololgy 1996;155:1604-1608.

Bals-Pratsch, M, Yoo YD, Knuth VA, Nieschlag E . Transdermal testosterone Substitution Therapy for male hypogonadism. Lancet 1986;4/943-946.

Brocks DR, Meikle AW, Boike SC, Mazer NA, Zariffa N, Audet PR, Jorkasky DK. Pharmacokinetics of testosterone in hypogonadal men after transdermal delivery: influence of dose. J Clinical Pharmacology 1996

Aug;36(8):732-9.

Carey PO, Howards SS, Vance ML. Transdermal testosterone treatment of hypogonadal men. Urology 1988 Jul;140(1):76-9.

Cutter CB. Compounded Percutaneous Testosterone Gel: Use and Effects in Hypogonadal Men. J American Board Family Practice 2001;14(1):22-32.

English KM, et al. Low-dose transdermal testosterone therapy improves angina threshold in men with chronic stable angina. Circulation 2000;102:1906-11.

Findlay JC, Place V, Snyder PJ. Transdermal delivery of Testosterone. J. Clinical Endocrinolology Metab.1989; 64; 266-268.

Howell S, Shalet S. Testosterone deficiency and replacement. Horm Res 2001;56 Suppl 1:86-92.

Kenny AM, et al. Effects of transdermal testosterone on lipids and vascular reactivity in older men with low bioavailable testosterone levels. J Gerontol A Biol Sci Med Sci 2002 Jul;57(7):M460-65.

Mazer NA. New clinical applications of transdermal testosterone delivery in men and women. J Control Release 2000 Mar 1;65(1-2):303-15.

McGriff-Lee NJ. Transdermal testosterone gel (Cellegy). Curr Opin Investig Drugs 2002 Nov;3(11):1629-32.

McNicholas TA, et al. A novel testosterone gel formulation normalizes androgen levels in hypogonadal men, with improvements in body composition and sexual function. Brit J. Urology International. 2003 Jan;91(1):69-74.

Shifren JL, et al. Transdermal testosterone treatment in women with impaired sexual function after oophorectomy. N Engl J Med. 2000 Sep 7;343(10):682-8. janshifren@hotmail.com

Sitruk-Ware R. Transdermal delivery of steroids. Contraception 1989 Jan;39(1):1-20

Wang C, et al. Pharmacokinetics of a transdermal gel in hypogonadal men .application of gel at one sit versus four sites : a General Clinical Research Center Study. J Clin Endocrinol Metab 2000 Mar;85(3):964-9.

Winters SJ, Atkinson L. Serum LH concentrations in hypogonadal men during transdermal testosterone replacement through scrotal skin: further evidence that ageing enhances testosterone negative feedback. Clin Endocrinol (Oxf). 1997 Sep;47(3):317-22.

Winters SJ. Current status of testosterone replacement therapy in men. Arch Fam Med. 2000 Mar;9(3):221. winters@med1.dept-med.pitt.edu

Viagra, ED and Testosterone

Aversa A, Isidori AM, Spera G, Lenzi A, Fabbri A. Androgens improve cavernous vasodilation and response to sildenafil in patients with erectile dysfunction. Clin Endocrinol (Oxf). 2003 May;58(5):632-8.

Basar M, et al. The efficacy of sildenafil in different etiologies of erectile dysfunction (ED). International Urol Nephrol. 2001;32(3):403-7.

Becker AJ, et al. Cavernous and systemic testosterone levels in different phases of human penile erection. Urology. 2000 Jul;56(1):125-9.

Chatterjee R, et al. Management of ED by combination therapy with testosterone and sildenafil in recipients of high-dose therapy for haematological malignancies. Bone Marrow Transplant. 2002 Apr;29(7):607-10.

Gauthier A, et al. Relative Efficacy of Sildenafil Compared to Other Treatment Options for Erectile Dysfunction South Med J 2000;93(10):962-965.

Guay AT, et al. Efficacy and safety of sildenafil citrate for treatment of erectile dysfunction in a population with associated organic risk factors. J Androl. 2001 Sep-Oct;22(5):793-7.

Lugg JA, Rajfer J, Gonzalez-Cadavid NF. Dihydrotestosterone is the active androgen in the maintenance of nitric oxide-mediated penile erection in the rat. Endocrinology 1995 Apr;136(4):1495-501.

Lim PH, Moorthy P, Benton KG. The clinical safety of Viagra. Ann N Y Acad Sci. 2002 May;962:378-88.

Manecke RG, Mulhall JP. Medical treatment of erectile dysfunction. Ann Med. 1999 Dec;31(6):388-98.

McCullough AR, et al. Achieving treatment optimization with sildenafil citrate (Viagra) in patients with erectile dysfunction. Urology. 2002 Sep;60(2 Suppl 2):28-38.

Reiter WJ, et al. Dehydroepi androsterone in the treatment of erectile dysfunction: a prospective, double-blind, randomized, placebo-controlled study. Urology 1999 Mar;53(3):590-4; discussion 594-5.

Shabsigh R. Hypogonadism and erectile dysfunction: the role for testosterone therapy. Int J Impot Res. 2003 Aug;15 Suppl 4:S9-13.

Shabsigh R. The effects of testosterone on the cavernous tissue and erectile function. World J Urol. 1997;15(1):21-6.

Steers W, Guay AT, et al. Assessment of the efficacy and safety of Viagra (sildenafil citrate) in men with ED. Int J Impotence Res. 2001 Oct;13(5):261-7.

Svetec DA, et al. The effect of parenteral testosterone replacement on prostate specific antigen in hypogonadal men with erectile dysfunction. J Urol 1997 Nov;158(5):1775-7.

INDEX

ACKNOWLEDGMENTS

My special thanks to Dr. Andre Guay, director of the Lahey Sex Clinic at Harvard, for his helpful suggestions and recent determination of the age-related ranges for testosterone. Several female physicians—Jeanne Alexander, Lorraine Dennerstein, Jennifer and Laura Berman, Lisa Tenover, Adrian Dobs, Leslie Lundt and Susan Davis—contributed to this manuscript by publishing their writings and research regarding male hormones and their role in women's sexual function. I am grateful to Dr. Lundt for her feedback and suggestions regarding brain chemistry.

Many ordinary people contributed to this manuscript with stories of their personal experiences when visiting doctors to ask about their sexual problems. Of course, I have obscured identifying details and combined features from several cases, but each and every patient supplied an integral aspect of the hormone experience. A variety of men who have written and visited me after reading my first book, *Listen To Your Hormones,* gave me a personal insight into dealing with these difficult issues.

The Endocrine Society meeting on endocrine disruptive chemicals and consultation with my colleagues provided useful background material for this book. I am very grateful to Andrew Weil and John Robbins for their clear perception of the ever-changing world of nutrition and its effect on healthy aging. I urge you to read their new books for their innovative recommendations.

I honor those researchers who have done all the hard work and developed their unique concepts in genetics, human sexuality, sleep disorders and neuropsychiatry. John Manning, Jeff Bowles, Dennis McFadden, Steven Krimsky, Theo Colborn, Deborah Cadbury, Joe Thornton, Meir Kryger and Owen Wolkowitz, are all great scientists and innovators in their own right.

CONTACT INFORMATION

To contact the doctor or to make comments or ask questions about the book, please write to Dr. Kryger, 1084 Cass Street, Suite B, Monterey, CA 93940, or email him at: drk@wellnessmd.com and please use www.Kryger. medem.com for confidential, secure email consultations.

Coming soon...
What will happen when medicine finally cures the major causes of death and disease—cancer, heart disease and diabetes? What will happen to the millions of baby boomers who are going to live beyond a century? Are humans really going to live longer and better lives? What if chronic diseases were "curable"? In Medicine we talk about cure, but we are a lot closer to this incredible goal than you might imagine. Curing diabetes has been an elusive dream for millions of diabetics. Now, thanks to nutritional genomics, it may be possible to do something about curing diabetes and reversing obesity.

According to a *Time* article in January 2005, "the promise of nutritional genomics is to understand on the most basic level how health is determined by the interplay of nutrients and genes. Medicine, science, genetics and technology can now join forces with powerful hormones to provide a treatment to help reverse obesity.

A new book written in conjunction with Dr. Gary Matson, a weight loss specialist from Fresno, California is on its way:

To be notified when Dr. Kryger's forthcoming controversial book about nutritional genomics becomes available, call: 831-373-4406, fax: 831-373-4481 or contact:

Abraham Kryger, MD, DMD
WellnessMD Publications
1084 Cass Street, Monterey, California 93940
Email the office at: WMDmgr@mbay.net or
DrK@WellnessMD.com

Dr. Kryger's first book, *Listen To Your Hormones,* published in 2004, is available at www.sexlove andhormones.com

ABOUT THE AUTHOR

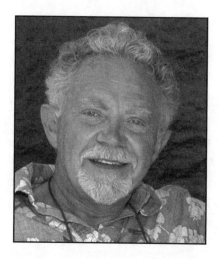

Dr. Abraham (Harvey) Kryger, a wellness pioneer, has been at the forefront of research in human hormone therapy, nutrition and preventive medicine for nearly three decades. He earned an MD and a DMD from the University of Manitoba in Canada. He has served for twenty years as Medical Director of the Monterey Preventive Medical Clinic and was formerly director of the Alternative Medicine Foundation in Santa Rosa and Marina, California. A board-certified Family Practitioner and Preventive Medicine specialist, Dr. Kryger operates a full-time private practice in Monterey, California.

Dr.Kryger's research credits include groundbreaking work in the use of phytopneutrient supplements to boost the immune system and help fight viral infections. He was awarded a patent for Testocreme®, a soy-based bio-identical testosterone used to restore men's libido, vitality and well-being. He has been interviewed on *Spotlight on Health* at "www.USAToday.com" and maintains three health information websites at "www.wellnessmd. com," "www.estocreme.com" and "www.testocreme.com" to build aware-ness of men's and women's health issues.